SIGNATURE ENERGY WORK

Accessing, Evaluating, and Transforming the Personal Energy Field

Copyright © 2005 Dr. Cora B. Llera, D.C.

10-Digit ISBN 1-59113-735-7
13-Digit ISBN 978-1-59113-735-1

All rights reserved. No part of this publication may be reproduced, stored in a retrieval system, or transmitted in any form or by any means, electronic, mechanical, recording or otherwise, without the prior written permission of the author.

Printed in the United States of America.

The author of this book does not prescribe the use of any technique as a form of treatment for physical, psychological or medical problems without the advice of a physician, either directly or indirectly. The intent of the author is only to offer information of a general nature. In the event you use any of the information in this book for yourself, which is your constitutional right, the author assumes no responsibility for your actions.

Booklocker.com, Inc.
2005

SIGNATURE ENERGY WORK

*Accessing, Evaluating, and Transforming
the Personal Energy Field*

Dr. Cora B. Llera, D.C.

CONTENTS

INTRODUCTION vii
CHAPTER 1 A SHIFTING PARADIGM 1
CHAPTER 2 A SIMPLE PATHWAY THROUGH THE
  PARADIGM 16
CHAPTER 3 WALKING THE PATHWAY 30
CHAPTER 4 SIGNATURE ENERGY WORK 35
CHAPTER 5 STEP ONE: IDENTIFY THE CORE
  QUESTION 39
CHAPTER 6 STEP TWO: FIND THE ANSWER 52
CHAPTER 7 STEP THREE: WORK WITH THE ENERGY 94
CHAPTER 8 WORKING THE LEVELS 116
CHAPTER 9 WORKING THE SIX W'S 135
CHAPTER 10 THE QUALITY OF WHY 178
CHAPTER 11 STEP FOUR -- RE-TEST 183
CHAPTER 12 STEP FIVE: THE EPILOGUE -
  PROCESSING, HOMEWORK, AND REFERRALS 185
NOTES 188
APPENDIX A: "O-RING" TESTING 193
APPENDIX B: FUNNEL TESTING 195
APPENDIX C: SURROGATE AND SELF-TESTING 196

APPENDIX D: GROUNDING AND CONNECTING 197
APPENDIX E: WHY PROCESSING 200
APPENDIX F: SEWLINE 202
APPENDIX G: SEWLINE REPORT OF FINDINGS 204
RESOURCES 206

INTRODUCTION

The purpose of this book is two-fold. The first is to present you with information that will direct you toward a new paradigm in healing work, be it professional work as a health-care provider, or your own personal healing work as an individual. The second is to provide you with a simple pathway to follow in your exploration of this new paradigm.

The old paradigm, which is represented by our mainstream Western medical system, views the human body as a closed mechanical system. Illness and disease, pain and problems are caused by something that is separate from the human "machine", and affects the machine from the outside "world". Solutions for problems, and cures for illnesses, are to be found outside of the human system. Treatment is performed "on" or administered "to" us, and we are passive recipients. This is an external path toward healing, in that both the cause of the problem and the tools for the cure come from "out there".

The new paradigm includes an internal path, based on the view that the human body is part of an open system that includes the mind. The mind consists of a conscious, intelligent field of energy that extends beyond the realm of material reality, and is not measurable by standards of time, mass, and space. The mind interacts with the human body via the brain. Illness and problems can originate at any level of the body-mind, and solutions are actively created from within our body-mind. The internal tools for creating solutions are consciousness and choice.

Signature Energy Work is the result of my own exploration of the new paradigm. It is a pathway toward healing that combines the external path and the internal, with the intention of forming a whole that is greater than the some of its parts, in which the two integrated paths complement and amplify each other. Signature

Energy Work employs muscle-testing (a simple yes-no questioning mechanism), in combination with the SEWLINE (a framework of exploratory questions), to access the intelligence of the body-mind. The information gleaned is then integrated with energy-work techniques to create a healing treatment. I will discuss each of these three tools—muscle-testing, the SEWLINE, and energy-work techniques—in detail, as they are the basic components of Signature Energy Work.

Signature Energy Work is the product of my 20 years of clinical experience imposed on the background of 40-plus years of life experience and spiritual and philosophical study. This book is meant as a teaching tool for the professional healer as well as the individual lay person to learn Signature Energy Work: to examine it, understand it, and master it. However, just as Signature Energy Work itself is the integration of all of my healing experiences and philosophies, I encourage you to use it as a starting point for the examination of your own healing background, beliefs, and interests, and then create your own healing pathway. Healing is a creative process; it's an art. Master the technical structure of any healing modality, and you become a technician. Stand on that structure and leap from it into the unknown, and you become an artist.

CHAPTER 1

A SHIFTING PARADIGM

"There's a way to solve every dilemma...Check your premises."
*- Francisco D'Anconia (*from Ayn Rand's *Atlas Shrugged)*

CASE STUDY #1 – NANCY
    I had actually known Nancy for years before her accident; I was her chiropractor, so she would come to me for an occasional adjustment to relieve a kink in her neck, or an ache in her back. In spite of these complaints - which she usually dismissed as the normal consequences of a busy life - Nancy always came in with a smile. She would greet everyone with a bright and enthusiastic hello, her robust energy as contagious as her humor and her optimism. After a visit with Nancy, *I* usually felt better.
    As she sits down in front of me now, however, she looks like it hurts just to think. I ask her how she's doing and she hesitates, as if searching for the energy to respond in her usual Nancy-way. She answers dully, repeating last week's response: her neck and back are fine, but she still has headaches. It doesn't take much to see that she's got a bad one today. When they come—and lately they've been coming daily—these headaches seem to absolutely drain her. In the six weeks since her accident they have gradually eroded her natural vitality and left her fatigued, irritable, and discouraged.
    Nancy had a car accident. It was a relatively minor rear-end collision, where she sustained a moderate whiplash injury: a strain to the muscles and ligaments of the neck and upper back, with a resulting distortion of the normal alignment of the vertebrae in that

area. I've been treating her intensely since then with chiropractic adjustments, massage therapy, and neuromuscular trigger point therapy—pretty standard chiropractic fare for this type of injury—and her neck and back pain have responded beautifully, receding gradually and steadily. But her headaches keep returning, with no significant diminution in their intensity or frequency. Each visit her normally hearty energy seems a little paler, slower, more fragile. Her x-rays, taken at the hospital after the accident, didn't show any evidence of fracture or pathology in the neck or back, and she actually didn't sustain any trauma to the head itself. There is no evidence of disc herniation or nerve impingement, and her family doctor has ruled out any systemic reason for her continuing headaches. There just seems to be no logical reason for her to be in so much pain. It's evident, however, that she is.

I ask her to lie down, and she heaves herself on to my treatment table with a punctuating sigh. She's not a small person, Nancy, partly because of her Central American Indian heritage, and partly because of years of hard work. When she came to this country, young and alone with 2 small children, her lack of education pushed her to work in a series of jobs that required a lot of physical labor, always for little pay. Because she was raising her kids on her own, she often worked two jobs at a time. She is currently employed as a nanny, caring long hours for a little boy whose mother left, and whose father is struggling to raise his young son while trying to run a small business. As she relaxes on the table, Nancy closes her eyes, takes a few deep breaths, and waits for me to begin the treatment.

I slide my hands under the back of her head, pressing my fingers under the ridge of the skull where the muscles of the neck and upper back converge onto the bone. Just being touched where it hurts helps her to relax even more, and I relax a little, too. This is one of the humbling moments in a doctor's life, when you have no reasonable idea what is wrong with, or what to do for your patient. I have given up many times at this point, telling the patient that I don't know what else I can do for them, and losing them to long-term pain medication or chronic illness. Losing a patient is never comfortable, and that is exactly what has pushed me to know more. It has taken me a long time, but what I have learned is the *value* of not knowing.

As I focus on my own deepening breath, I feel the familiar sense of expansion and connection that comes with touch. It's like a wave of compassion that hits me, and then rolls through me and outward toward my patient, filling the room with a deep silence, a reverence, a profound sense of focus. I settle into the moment gratefully. As difficult a journey as it has been for me to arrive at this moment, I am thankful, if not for the struggle, then certainly for its fruits. This is the moment of not knowing; of surrendering into that which allows me to move past the limitations of the known, and into the finer vibrations of the yet-to-be-known.

Departure from the External Path

This moment represents my departure from the modern western medical model in which I was trained: the practice of medicine based exclusively on the tenets of objectivism, founded on the idea that *consciousness* (the rational mind) *perceives reality*. Objective medicine requires an objective, measurable analysis of the physical mechanism being analyzed, and excludes any consideration of consciousness in this object. The objective observer and the observed are separate and unrelated, and it is the job of the observer to rationally perceive the unchanging nature of the observed. Earth scientist Gregg Braden calls this approach to healing the path of "external technology,"[1] in which both the cause and the cure for illness or discomfort is assumed to come from outside of the patient, from somewhere "out there." Disease, deficiency, and injury are something that *happens* to us, and their cure is found through things that we do for the *condition*: drugs, dietary supplements, surgery, even chiropractic manipulation. Mind you, the external technology of modern medicine is something that has proven highly successful and beneficial for many, including myself. This approach, however, requires that I see myself as separate from my patient, both emotionally and physically, which would seem to discourage both touch and empathy. Years of clinical practice have proven to me that an objective physical examination of my patient is both necessary and valuable, but the information it provides is limited. In addition, my experience has shown me that a diagnosis and treatment based solely on objective modalities provides limited results. The proof is in Nancy, who has had a thorough and objective physical examination by three different physicians, has had access to all the available treatments that modern medicine can offer, and yet still has unexplained headaches.

The path of external technology-based medicine has risen from the science of Sir Isaac Newton. The Newtonian model of physical reality views the world as a huge clocklike machine, with interconnecting parts that each have their own separate function, and work together in a precise manner—like "clockwork." The modern medical system views the human body in much the same way, as a complex biomechanical structure of inert matter—bones, muscles, nerves, organs, etc.—that acts according to a predictable, linear pattern, unrelated to the influence of consciousness or creativity. Modern medical practitioners (and I must reiterate that as a modern chiropractic physician, I fall into this category) approach the treatment of their patients as a clockmaker approaches repairing a clock: first, inspect it to determine which part is not working, and then adjust, clean, repair, or replace said part.

At this moment I am starkly aware that the reductionist Newtonian model of medicine, and therefore the scope of my traditional professional training and knowledge, has taken me—and my patient—as far as it can. There's nothing left but to admit that I don't know what is causing Nancy's headaches. The fact that none of her other doctors seem to know either is soothing to my ego, but it's not helping Nancy. It's clearly time to take a broader look at the problem, and this necessitates including the subjective viewpoint, my own as well as Nancy's. Obviously the traditional chiropractic therapy that I've been performing has given her temporary relief, which is probably what has kept her coming to me, but temporary relief becomes expensive, and eventually it just becomes discouraging. It's really no way to live. It's my willingness to *not* know what Nancy needs, to recognize the limitations of my objective knowledge, that allows me to relax my ego, expand outward beyond the limits of my five senses—beyond the limitations of objective physical reality—and connect to the subjective.

Subjective Reality – The Internal Path

"There is no objective reality!"[2] according to Dr. Candace Pert, the biophysicist who researched how our thoughts and emotions affect our health. She points out that our brains can only assimilate so much sensory information at one time: left without some kind of filtering system for the constant barrage of sensory stimulus coming at us from all sides, our brains would quickly go into overload, with mental chaos as the result. The system for filtering information from our environment is our emotions. Our emotions prioritize what information is important to us, and what can safely be ignored. As a result, our perception of reality, our personal understanding of "truth," is constantly being modified and interpreted through the organizing structure of our emotions. The objective scientific "truth" of Newtonian physics is based on the idea that there is only one truth, which can be objectively measured, and whose measurements can be replicated experimentally. The discoveries of modern quantum physics, however, show that the measurer himself influences the outcome of every experimental measurement he performs, by virtue of his own unique subjective observation of the experiment, and his measurements.

Our subjective aspect extends well beyond the mechanistic world of Newtonian science, and into this "quantum realm" of modern physics. As Stephen Hawking, the eminent quantum physicist of our time says, "…apparently common sense notions work well when dealing with material things like apples and/or comparatively slow moving things like planets; they don't work at all for things moving at the speed of light." [3] Such as thoughts, emotions, information. The quantum realm is the realm of thought and emotion, the realm of pure energy, where everything is still held in potential, and nothing has yet congealed into form. Our subjective aspect is the aspect of our selves that is fluidly connected to all energy, all knowledge, and all potential. It's the realm of the mind, the higher self, spirit, soul. It is the realm where consciousness *creates* reality.

The Quantum Realm

A *quantum* is defined as a "discrete quantity of electro-magnetic radiation,"[4] and "the lowest denomination of energy."[5] As the physicists who followed Newton studied the nature of matter, they focused on progressively smaller parts in a search for the essential building block of matter, eventually reaching the level of subatomic particles. They found that as the particles get smaller, they move faster; eventually the smallest subatomic particles approach the speed of light. And this is where things get interesting. At these extreme high speeds, the particles take on the characteristics of light. A quantum, then, is a subatomic particle that is essentially a very short burst of light (an extremely fast electromagnetic vibration) that contains a small byte of information. Albert Einstein theorized (in his Unified Field Theory[6]), and quantum physicists have demonstrated, that our entire world consists of these bursts of light clinging together, rapidly firing in synchronized groups, to form fields of light that appear to our eyes as something solid, very similar to how a digital photograph is formed by tiny pixels coming together to form a picture. Our physical world, then, is created by the actions of these nonphysical light/information particles gathering together into fields, vibrating at different speeds; the slower vibrating fields appear denser, like rocks and metal, the faster vibrations appear as living things like plants and people, the really fast vibrations make up non-physical things like radio waves, vibrating so fast that our eyes can't see them.

Researchers have extensively (and objectively) studied non-physical human energy fields - the electro-magnetic energy fields associated with the human body—using measurements taken with specialized electronic equipment.[7] Physiologist Valerie Hunt found that every material substance, living or inanimate, has a unique field of energy surrounding it that vibrates at its own unique vibratory level, what Dr. Hunt calls the "vibratory signature"[8] of an object. The human energy field has been measured at a range of vibratory levels, some as high as 200,000 cycles per second.[9] The lower levels of vibration in the human energy field are associated with the physical structure of the body: the cells, bones, organs, etc. In fact, Gregg Braden noted that each organ of the human body has its own distinctive vibrational frequency, what he calls the "signature frequency"[10] of the organs:

for example, a healthy human heart resonates at a signature frequency of about 7.8 Hertz. (Interestingly enough, Braden, in his work as an earth scientist and engineer, pointed out that the equivalent signature frequency of the planet Earth is also 7.8 Hertz.) The higher levels of vibration in the human energy field are associated with the non-physical aspects of the human being, what Hunt calls the "mind-field" – the energy field of the mind.

Quanta, these bursts of light/information that are the basis for everything—human mind as well as human body—have not only a particle nature, but also a wave nature. As I understand it (and with my apologies to all quantum physicists out there), quanta hang out in waves, what physicists call waves of possibility. A quantum is like a single picture. A bunch of unrelated or non-sequential pictures aren't much good, so the pictures tend to arrange themselves in a certain order of appearance that form something like a movie—a wave of pictures. The pictures, if directed by some sort of intelligence, could be rearranged into an infinite number of movies, just by bringing them together in a different order. So the "waves of possibility" are possible movies formed by the arrangement and rearrangement of these pictures. All movies are a possibility, until someone decides to bring the pictures together to form a particular one: to change a possibility into a reality. Or, in the language of physicist Amit Goswami, "Quantum objects exist as a superposition of possibilities until our observation brings about actuality from potentiality, one actual, localized event from the many potential events."[11]

So who brings the pictures together to form a particular movie? We do, merely by *observation*. "Quantum possibilities do not become actuality until we, sentient beings, look at them and choose."[12] We actually do, according to the laws of physics, create our own reality. We choose a possibility from the quantum realm—where all possibilities are milling around, talking amongst themselves, so to speak—and the possibilities "collapse" from the quantum realm into the physical realm. Energy coalesces into form—the pictures come together to form a movie.

And how do we choose a possibility? With our brain. Or, more exactly, with our mind.

Human Mind: Human Body

In the external technological view of conventional Western medicine, the brain and the mind are one and the same. Until recently, science has told us that the mind is contained within the physical structure of the brain, but philosophers and healers have been positing for centuries that the mind goes far beyond the physical body. The ancient Greeks—Pythagoras, Plato, and Socrates, among others—commented about the exact nature and location of the mind. In ancient China, the Taoist view presented the brain as merely a physical organ through which the human mind—the temporal aspect of the formless, boundless, immortal primordial spirit—exerts control over the body. According to Daniel Reid, a practitioner of Chinese medicine and author of multiple books on the subject, "Primordial spirit is formless, boundless, and immortal, but in order to function in the temporal material world it must manifest a temporal aspect, which is called the 'human mind', including emotions and thoughts...The brain is a two-way terminal by which the mind exerts command over the body, and the state of the body influences the state of the mind."[13] The Chinese originated the idea that mind and body create each other, a concept that gave rise to the term coined by author Diane Connelly: bodymind. This is the integration of the external and internal paths, and implies what quantum physics confirms, that *consciousness creates reality through perception.*

According to the ancient Hawaiians (in their psycho-religious system, called Huna)[14], the physical body and brain are both controlled by non-physical intelligences: by both a "lower self" and a "middle self." The lower self is the intelligence of the physical body; it services the needs of the body based on non-logical, survival-imperative thinking, similar to the "subconscious mind" of modern psychology. The middle self is a non-physical intelligence that takes up temporary residence in the physical body, as the guest of the lower self, and regulates thoughts and feelings based on the logical thinking of the "conscious mind"—the human mind. The Kahuna, the ancient Hawaiian practitioners of Huna, believed that our lower and middle selves also interact with a non-physical "Higher Self." The Higher Self employs conceptual thinking, insight, and imagination to govern what psychologist Abraham Maslow called our "meta needs"[15]: the need for truth, beauty, wisdom, justice, and humor—our spiritual needs. The Higher Self is equivalent to the "superconscious mind," or what Valerie Hunt calls the "Infinite Mind": the mind of the cosmos.

Hunt sees the human mind and the cosmic mind like "two massive holographic computers," each holding the reservoirs of information and experience of man and the universe, respectively. Neurophysicist Karl Pribram explored the idea that the human mind contains a memory hologram—a memory bank of *all* human memory, sometimes referred to as *collective reality*[16]: the collection of all human consciousness. Pribram eventually won a Nobel Prize for the idea. Physicist David Bohm described a similar memory-hologram for the universe, containing the memory of every physical event that has occurred in the universe.[18] And experimental physicist/engineer Bob Beck found that when tuned to a specific brain wave frequency (at approximately 7.8 cycles per second), the human mind hologram actually interfaces with the cosmic mind hologram.[19] The concept of a human-cosmic interface is nearly identical to the ancient Hawaiians belief that the lower and middle selves—the human brain and the human mind—interact with the Higher Self. Dr. Candace Pert confirmed, in her research at the National Institutes of Health, that the physical brain is not the director of information to the body, but merely a receiver of information from the mind. She found that the brain is just one more stop on "a vast superhighway of internal information exchange taking place on a molecular level."[20] In other words, the mind networks with the brain *and* the body, communicating at a molecular level via a vast messenger system of peptides and peptide receptor sites throughout the body. Pert contends that the intelligence that directs the brain (the intelligence that is the human mind) originates in the non-physical realm. Because information has an unlimited capacity for expansion, "it cannot belong to the material world we apprehend with our senses, but must belong to its own realm, one that we can experience as emotion, the mind, the spirit—*an inforealm!*"[21] Others call this "inforealm" the mind-field, the quantum realm, the quantum self.

If the intelligence of the mind is what creates matter, if our human consciousness indeed creates our reality, based on our perceptions, then why, you may ask, don't we seem to be *aware* that we are creating our reality while we're creating it? If our reality truly *is* a matter of choice, surely many of us would choose a different reality!

Again according to Goswami, we don't often find ourselves in a state of consciousness that encourages us to choose freely. "It happens when we are creative, for example, when we experience deep compassion for another being, when we get moral insights, or when we are in communion with nature…I call [such a state] the quantum self because of its connection with the complete freedom of choice in quantum measurement."[22] Our sense of self in this state is expansive. It goes beyond the normal personal boundaries of our ego, and seems to encompass, and unite us with, the universe.

The trick, then, to choosing a reality that is not based solely on the perceptions of our ego—that is, on our fears, our conditioning, or our past—is to choose from a higher state of awareness, from the level of the q*uantum self*. This is the level of perception where the human mind and the cosmic mind interface, where the lower and middle selves communicate with the Higher Self. It's the state that I attempt to access in Signature Energy Work.

Valerie Hunt states that, "Ultimate reality is contacted not through the physical sense of the material world, but through deep intuition...Living is a transaction, an interaction with other force fields, with an element of choice. This is a domain beyond time, space, and mass where only vibrations exist."[23]

NANCY (continued)

I break into the relaxed silence between us, by telling Nancy that I believe—and I emphasize the words "*I* believe" so that she understands that this is my own frame of reference, and that she doesn't have to buy it—that the human being is much more than what meets the eye. In fact the physical aspects of the human being—the parts we can see—are just the tip of the iceberg. Scientific research, I explain, indicates that we humans are composed of physical, as well as mental, emotional, and spiritual aspects, and that these aspects inter-relate. This means that for every physical condition we experience, like headaches, there is the potential for an equally important emotional, mental, or even spiritual level of cause for that condition. I point out to Nancy that, until now, we have been working only on the physical level of her condition, and that her neck and back pain have completely resolved with that. But not her headaches. I suggest that perhaps her headaches have more to them than just the physical, and that in order to make more progress, we need to explore the other levels.

I use the analogy of the physical body as a lamp. Some lamps are prettier than others, some bigger, some brighter, but all lamps are designed to plug into an energetic system, wherein, if we flip the switch to the lamp, it should light up. (The lamp is part of an *electrical* energy system, whereas the physical body is part of a much more multidimensional energy system, but the relationships between the body/lamp and their respective energy systems are similar.) When we flip the light-switch and nothing happens, or the lamp shines only dimly, this is an indication that something is wrong, although the problem is not necessarily with the lamp itself. The problem may just as likely be somewhere else in the electrical system. I believe that Nancy's headaches, like any illness, are her body's way of trying to get her attention, to tell her that something is wrong. I believe that pain is our body sounding an alarm, indicating the need for change. Sometimes there *is* something wrong with the lamp—change is needed only at a physical level, like adjusting the spine or changing our diet. But it's just as likely that the problem is not with the lamp but the wiring, or perhaps the fuse—the change needs to be at another level of the electrical system. We can make alterations on any level: at the emotional level, by changing how we deal with our feelings; at the mental level, by changing beliefs and ideas; or at the spiritual level, by altering how we pursue the themes and purposes of our life.

Pain and illness are not our body betraying us, but rather attempting to assist us in growing. If we look at it that way, we can work *with* the pain, rather than resist it. If we trust that our body is trying to communicate with us, rather than hurt us, we will listen to it. It has been my experience, in 20 years of listening to bodies, that when we get the message, the body stops sounding the alarm.

Nancy nods her head. Perhaps she's just too tired to question my explanation, but it looks like she's following me, so far. We know that Nancy's headaches mean that a problem exists, we just haven't found out where in the system the problem is located. Is the light bulb burned out, or the wiring frayed? Is the lamp plugged in? Is there power to the switch?

I explain that beyond our physical body—through which we see, touch, smell and hear—lie the emotional, mental and spiritual bodies; collectively known as the "energy body". This is the system of energy that surrounds our physical body, and is invisible to the naked eye. It contains all of our thoughts and beliefs, is organized by our emotions, and is directly connected to the power source for our potential and our purpose. This multidimensional system, or "field," of energy is like the house that surrounds, and is connected to, the lamp. Our physical body lies within the energy body, and is constantly influenced by its energies. And because these energies are not in physical form, they fluctuate and change as our thoughts, feelings, and self-understanding changes. In addition, these energies have an effect on the people who come into contact with our field; anyone who enters our house is influenced by its ambiance. Research indicates that the human energy field extends anywhere from a few inches to several feet away from our physical body[24], so anyone who comes within a few feet of us has entered our energetic "home". Just as the lighting and color and furniture arrangement in each room of our home creates a distinct feeling for anyone who enters, each of our thoughts and beliefs, each of our habitual emotional reactions gives off its own characteristic energy frequency. Anyone who enters our energy field can feel it. These signature frequencies can be measured scientifically, and can be seen psychically. The sum total of all of the electromagnetic signatures of every thought, feeling, and belief that we have ever had, as well as the signature frequencies of every organ, tissue, cell, and molecule in our physical structure, are what make up our energy field. You can easily see that the result is a distinctly different energetic pattern for each human being, a pattern as unique as our fingerprint or our handwriting. This overall pattern is what identifies us as individuals; it's our signature in the universal language of energy. I call it our signature energy.

SIGNATURE ENERGY WORK

Nancy looks at me thoughtfully. Lately she's been very uncomfortable in her energetic home, especially in the room that is her head.

CHAPTER 2

A SIMPLE PATHWAY THROUGH THE PARADIGM

"The best description of healing refers to the activation of the body's energies toward dynamic equilibrium, growth, and evolution."
Dr. Valerie V. Hunt

The Structure of the Human Energy Field

From the simplest form of matter to the most complex cosmic event, everything is composed of light/ information/vibration organized into fields of energy. Energetic fields, whether biological or cosmic, have an internal organization that allows each field to interact with other fields. Dr. Valerie Hunt's research demonstrated that human energy fields have a range of frequencies. The extremely low frequency fields are associated with basic human biological processes, and the patterns of these low frequency fields are similar for all humans. Each molecule in our bodies gives off an electromagnetic field, as does each cell, tissue, and organ. A liver cell gives off a different frequency of field than does a kidney cell, but all healthy liver cells give the same characteristic frequency in all people.

The extremely high frequency human energy fields are associated with the mind, and higher levels of awareness. Hunt concluded that the patterns of these high frequency human energy fields are not at all similar from one person to the next, in fact she found that each person's mind-field consisted of clusters of energy

SIGNATURE ENERGY WORK

interspersed with gaps along the frequency scale, forming a distinctive pattern of energy-cluster-to-gap that was absolutely unique for each person. The clumps of energetic output are associated with emotional states, and the pattern of habitual emotional states—what Hunt calls the individual emotional signature—are formed by the individual's responses to events and stimuli over the course of a lifetime, or even many lifetimes. Our emotional signature is what organizes our awareness into the unique vibratory pattern that is our human mind-field, and our human mind-field is what interfaces with the cosmic mind-field. The light/information that flows from the cosmic mind-field, channeled through our human mind-field, funnels down to our brain-body network to direct the formation of our physical reality. Our physical reality is formed, then, from our thoughts; and is shaped by our emotions. Energy precedes form.

    Healers and mystics from ancient and indigenous cultures—the ancient Hindu Vedic texts, the Kabbalah of mystic Judaism, the Tibetan, Indian, and Japanese Zen Buddhists, among many others—have spoken for centuries about energy, and the human energy field. John White, in his book *Future Science*[25], enumerates 97 different cultures that refer to the human energy field using 97 different names: aura, energy field, energy bodies, subtle bodies being just a few. Many cultures describe the makeup of the human energy field, and while the terms vary, the basic structure is almost universally described as being composed of levels, or layers, of energy expanding progressively farther outward from the physical, to form what looks like concentric shells of energy around the body. Barbara Brennan, a NASA research scientist, psychotherapist, and practicing healer, describes the layers of the human energy field, as well as the history of scientific investigation into the human energy field, in her book *Hands of Light: A Guide to Healing through the Human Energy Field*. Brennan has developed what she calls "high sense perception"—the ability to see higher vibrations of energy—and describes the human energy field as having layers composed of increasingly higher vibrational frequencies of energy – physical, emotional, mental, and spiritual energies. "Each succeeding layer interpenetrates completely all the layers under it, including the physical body...Actually, each body is not a 'layer' at all, although that is what we may perceive. It is, rather, a more expansive version of our self that carries within it the other, more limited forms."[26] Brennan explains that in order to perceive each level, the practitioner must raise his consciousness to each successively higher vibrational frequency level, the lowest level being the vibrations of the gross physical body, which we perceive through our five physical senses.

    The first *non*-physical level of the human energy field, according to Brennan, is called the *etheric* level, or *etheric body*. This layer sits closest to the physical body, and is associated with the autonomic functions of the physical body such as breathing, digestion, cellular growth and repair. The second layer is the *emotional* level, associated with feelings and emotional life, and the third layer is the *mental* level, associated with rational, linear thinking. These first three levels all process energies related to our physical world, and comprise what is commonly referred to as the mind, or more specifically, the personal human mind. Brennan describes a total of seven layers of the human energy field, and indicates that the upper three levels relate to the energies of the *spiritual* world – what I have referred to as the Universal (cosmic) mind, or quantum realm. The fourth level is the middle layer between the upper and lower three layers; it's the interface layer between the physical and spiritual worlds, or we could say, between the personal human mind and the Universal mind. Brennan states that this fourth layer processes the energy of love.

Evaluating the Individual Energy Field

The energy field of any individual can only be examined by taking into consideration all of the elements that contribute to their energetic signature: the entire storehouse of that person's emotions, thoughts, and spiritual beliefs. I contend that these less tangible aspects of the signature energy cannot be assessed accurately, if assessed only by the usual scientific objective means. After all, how am I to understand the feelings of my patient if I am prohibited from connecting with her emotionally, from engaging my own emotions? If I hold myself at an "objective distance" from my patient, how can I gain insight into what she believes, and the context for these beliefs? In assessing the truth about a patient, I must understand her truth, not just my truth about her. Parker J. Palmer, in his book, *The Courage to Teach*, states that the purely objective approach to knowledge is grounded in fear—fear that if we get too close to the thing we wish to examine (in this case, the true nature of my patient's problem), the "impure contents of our subjective lives will contaminate the thing and our knowledge of it."[27] We, as modern medical practitioners, are afraid to get too close to our patients—to touch them, listen to them, relate to them—because we are not comfortable with our own subjective nature. We are afraid of "contaminating" our patients with our own, subjective viewpoint. In addition, as individuals engaged in our own self-healing journey, we are afraid of being contaminated by the subjective viewpoint, the imperfect energy, of our patients. And finally, we are afraid, as individuals charged with the responsibility of creating our reality, of looking too deeply at the imperfection of our own signature energy.

Signature energy work requires the development of a method of knowing that takes into account the subjective energies of both doctor and patient: the observer and the observed. This subjective sense, the sixth sense, if you will, is what allows us to perceive the mind-field—the personal and collective human mind-field as well as the cosmic mind-field. In the standard medical world, the subjective is avoided, and even considered something to be overcome. The result is medicine in the masculine model, based on detachment, objectivity, a narrowing of focus on specific parts: the power of the intellect. Signature energy work is based on a more wholistic model, which *builds* on this masculine foundation and adds—rather than denies—the feminine mode of knowing, based on resonance, affinity, expansion of focus to encompass the whole: the power of empathy, compassion, and intuition.

Our fear of the "impure contents"[28] of our subjective perceptions is banished when we come to the table with the assumption that *all* of our perceptions are valuable, that both our objective *and* subjective perceptions contribute to our understanding of the whole – the whole patient: her physical being as well as her feelings, memories, and beliefs. By letting go of the assumption that our subjective perceptions can only "contaminate" the object of our assessment, an opening is created for interaction, an interaction between the subjective nature of the examiner and the examined, patient and doctor. By moving past the assumption that it is inappropriate for us to be open to our patients, to becoming willing to be changed by our interaction with them, a resonance is formed between the healer and the one who seeks to be healed. The phenomena of resonance[29] suggests that it is the affinity between the contents of my signature energy, and the contents of my patient's, that allows me to consciously identify her signature energy, and in the process, to become conscious of my own. In the resonant state, the thoughts, feelings, and physical sensations of the perceiver and the perceived add together, expanding the range of perception for both. If we allow all of our perceptions in this expanded state to have meaning, then we have created the experience of intuition.

NANCY (continued)

I explain to Nancy that while scientists have found ways to document and measure the signature energy, using sensitive and sophisticated electronic equipment, only those people who have a very well developed clairvoyance can actually *see* energy. I'm not one of those people, so I have created my own method for assessing the signature energy of my patients. I explain that I will use the same method of muscle-testing that, until now, I've been using to determine which vertebra or muscle group needs attention during her treatment. But this time I'll use the muscle-testing to find out how her signature energy might be involved with her headaches, and how best to work with the signature energy in order to eliminate her headaches. I reiterate that I'm going to be asking questions silently, using the strength and resistance of her hand muscle as a yes-or-no answer. But in addition to checking her spine, as she has experienced so often during the course of her chiropractic treatments, I am also going to test various reflex points on her head, neck, abdomen and legs, as well as some points that are actually off the body, in her energy field. I promise that I'll explain to her what I find, once I put it all together, and that all she needs to do now is hold the two fingers of her hand together in the usual "O-ring" configuration[30], and resist my attempts to pull open the "O".

Muscle-Testing: The Interface of Mind and Body

> "*The individual human mind is like a computer terminal connected to a giant database. The database is human consciousness itself, of which our own cognizance is merely an individual*

expression, but with its roots in the common consciousness of all mankind. This database is the realm of genius; because to be human is to participate in the database, everyone, by virtue of his birth, has access to genius. The unlimited information contained in the database has now been shown to be readily available to anyone in a few seconds, at any time and in any place. This is indeed an astonishing discovery, bearing the power to change lives, both individually and collectively, to a degree never yet anticipated."
Dr. David Hawkins[31]

Muscle-testing has been used for decades (if not longer) as a mechanism to determine subjective truth: a tool for accessing the "database" of human consciousness. The modern definitive study on muscle-testing was published in 1971 by three physical therapists, Kendall, Kendall, and Wadsworth.[32] A chiropractor, Dr. George Goodheart, developed his own work with muscle-testing into a system called Applied Kinesiology, in which he showed that the strength or weakness of each muscle in the body is associated with the function of a specific corresponding organ and acupuncture meridian. In 1976 Dr. Goodheart began teaching his work to his colleagues. I myself studied Applied Kinesiology in my chiropractic post-graduate classes. The techniques became popular with many types of holistic practitioners as a method to detect and treat disease, based on the clear demonstration that muscles become weak when exposed to stimuli that can cause disease in the corresponding organ system, and become stronger when exposed to therapeutic substances.

I have to admit that for about the first 9 years after I learned Applied Kinesiology, I didn't use it in my clinical practice. I really didn't believe it; it seemed impractically complex and, yes, unbelievably subjective. Then I came upon the work of Dr. John Diamond, a psychiatrist who used muscle-testing to diagnose and treat his patients in a system he called "behavioral kinesiology."[33] Dr. Diamond worked with psychological stimuli, using a simplified version of muscle-testing to study the effects on his patients. Dr. Diamond demonstrated that any muscle of the body will be instantly weakened by the presence of unhealthy emotional attitudes or mental stresses. This concept electrified me. It was a perfect explanation for why patients like Nancy don't respond to standard western medical treatments—to *my* treatments—and it transformed my dormant Applied Kinesiology training into a tool for exploring first-hand the mind-body concept: how my patients' emotional and mental patterns related to their physical complaints.

More recently, I found the writings of Dr. David Hawkins, a psychiatrist who conducted a 15 year-long study using muscle-testing, and reported his conclusions in his book, *Power vs. Force*. He found that a person's responses to muscle-testing are "completely independent" of the person's "…intellectual opinions, reason, or logic." [34] This study confirmed what I have experienced in my own practice: muscle-testing is a mechanism that can be used to ask questions beyond the conscious levels of the body-mind, the subconscious as well as the superconscious levels. I can, in effect, ask any question, and use the resistance of any normal muscle to provide an answer.

When I ask a question, I then test the resistance of a muscle to see if that muscle is "strong"—able to maintain resistance—or "weak" in response to my question. The strong response indicates a "yes" answer to my question, the weak response indicates "no." I ask questions silently so that the conscious mind has no chance to interfere with the answer. It is the energetic patterns that are held beyond the level of consciousness that are usually the reason behind illnesses that have no physical explanation. Bringing these patterns to our conscious awareness, and understanding how these patterns limit our growth, allows us to gain control of them: to choose differently.

Surrendering the Ego, Surrendering Doubt

The most difficult aspect of using muscle-testing in my practice, for me, is that muscle-testing not only circumvents the conscious mind of the patient as a source of information, but it also circumvents the practitioner's. The information accessed through muscle-testing is coming from beyond the conscious aspects of the patient; from beyond their intellect, and from beyond mine. In doing so, I am eliminating my individual ego, my limited knowledge and intellect, as the authority. That may sound easy, if a little new-agey, but wait until you try it.

If you are going to ask questions of the quantum realm via muscle testing, you have to accept the answers that you are given, *and act on them*. This requires a certain amount of humility (and/or desperation.) Having always been something of an intellectual snob, I found it very difficult to subordinate my intellect to the intelligence of the quantum realm; after all, I have college degrees! I had proudly—and successfully, thank-you-very-much—conducted my practice for years, relying on my training and my education; that is, on my well-developed ego. But patients like Nancy brought me inevitably up against the limits of my objective knowledge. Repeatedly. Only in the most desperate circumstances would I "resort" to muscle testing as a diagnostic tool. This became an annoyingly common cycle for me, and I did it again and again, each time just the tiniest bit less arrogantly than the last. Finally at some point I began to embrace the humility option, and started to trust the information that I got through muscle-testing. Actually, I started to notice that the information was correct. When I went with it, it worked. I gradually, *gradually*, trusted the quantum realm enough to actually use it out of choice, rather than need. I gradually learned to use muscle testing *first,* to access the quantum level, and then use my intelligence to help me interpret the information I received there. This step, as obvious as it sounds, was the hardest. It required wrestling down my self-doubt.

Doubt is the biggest obstacle to connecting with our quantum self, and self-doubt is the primary form. We are socialized from an early age to believe that we are incapable of surviving, or of being loved, just as we are. When we are young enough, we are, in fact, incapable of surviving alone, without the care and attention of those around us. We are dependent on our caregivers, so we learn how to please them: what to do, when, and how, in order to insure their love. In our minds, love and survival become inextricably linked, and neither one is guaranteed. We come to believe that we must be something else, something more than our natural selves, if we are to survive, which inevitably leads us to doubt what we are, what comes naturally to us. So we project a persona that is better—prettier, stronger, braver, in my case smarter—than we think we are in order to hide our inadequacy, in order to be loved, and in order to live. This "better" persona is our ego, and while it does, in fact, help us survive, it often gets out of hand. Especially as we become adults. As we come to rely on the ego, the mask of our "better self," we become so identified with it that we forget who we are. We start to think that we *are* the mask, that we *need* to be the mask; the ego dominates.

When the ego dominates, we spend the bulk of our lives trying to protect ourselves from our inherent weaknesses. In doing so, we cut ourselves off from our inherent strengths. Our natural gifts are left behind, unexplored and abandoned. Self-expression— the cultivation and expression of our gifts, our natural strengths— is squelched in favor of performance, the performance of the ego. Relying on muscle testing means relying on the truth that is revealed at the quantum level, the truth of our higher self, not our parents' truth, not our ego's truth. Relying on the truth of our quantum self means allowing the higher self to dominate, which forces the ego to surrender its constant doubt and to confront its relentless fear of not being enough. In our modern medical culture, where objective facts are valued, and the wisdom of the higher self is unacknowledged, this is asking a lot.

The Mechanics of Muscle-Testing

Kinesiologic testing can be performed on any muscle, and is often used as a diagnostic tool in orthopedic and neurological medicine to evaluate the level of weakness of an injured muscle, or a muscle innervated by a damaged nerve. In Signature Energy Work I choose a normal muscle to test with, using it as a tool to access and read the signature energy. Many kinesiologists muscle-test using a combination of arm muscles. I prefer to test on one single muscle at a time, and I usually like to use the adductor muscle of the thumb, the "O-ring" muscle, simply because it results in less work for both me and the patient during repetitive testing. Here is how it works:

1. I ask the patient to hold the tips of the thumb and pinkie finger of one hand together firmly, forming an "O" with the hand.
2. I test the normal strength of this muscle by attempting to pull these two fingers apart, using each of my own index fingers placed inside the "O" and pulling outward. Normally, the patient is able to maintain the "O" against my pull. This is the "yes" mode in my question/answer process.
3. I ask the patient to hold the "O" together, and then silently ask to be shown the "no" mode, while again

pulling outward on the patient's fingers with my own. A "no" answer is demonstrated by the patient's inability to sustain his thumb and pinkie held together against the pull of my fingers.

Muscle-testing should not be a life-and-death struggle, so I instruct my patient to hold his fingers together firmly against my resistance, but not to throw his whole body into it. My resistive pull is firm also, but not so firm that I am always pulling the patient's fingers apart. I will repeat the 3 steps above until I get a feel for a particular patient's muscle tension and strength, and I find the right amount of pull to use in order to get a consistently clean "yes" or "no" response on that patient. Everyone is different, so I have to be willing to play with it a little.

If my patient is not able to hold his fingers together, because of injury to the hand, overall weakness, inability to comprehend the muscle test mechanism, etc., or if I am unable to register a clear "yes" versus "no" response on the patient, I may choose another muscle to conduct my testing on, or I may move to surrogate testing. Surrogate testing can be performed by using another person to muscle-test, as a stand-in for the patient. I often use surrogate testing when examining small children: I ask an adult (usually the mother or father) to hold or embrace the child/patient while I muscle test using the adult's hand muscle, but asking questions about the child. This works well for two reasons: small children tend to be intimidated by strange doctors, and they are often too young, or too squirmy, to focus on sustaining a muscle-testing mode for more than a minute or so.

I also use myself as a surrogate for my patients when necessary. This requires mastering the fine art of muscle-testing on one's self. I usually self-surrogate like this:

1. Ask a yes-or-no question.

2. Form the "O" with thumb and pinkie-finger of the non-dominant hand (in my case, this is my left hand).
3. Use the thumb and index finger of the dominant (my right) hand to push apart the "O".
4. If I can push open the "O" with my other hand in response to a question, this is a "no" response to my question. If the "O" stays closed, this is a "yes". (Weak=no, Strong=yes)

Self-surrogate testing opens up another avenue of signature energy work: self-testing. This means using myself as a surrogate for myself. I can follow the 4 steps above, while asking questions about myself, as the patient. This moves me in a most interesting direction: self-healing, the exploration and repair of my own signature energy.

Compassion: Key to Intuition

Ah, you say! Didn't we establish earlier that muscle-testing bypasses the conscious mind, the intellect? And didn't I say that I always ask my muscle-testing questions silently, in order not to bias the conscious mind of my patient? Yes, indeed. Then how, you may ask, can I muscle-test on myself, without bias?

Sometimes I can't. Sometimes I can. What makes the difference between the two is neutrality. If I can be completely neutral, I can test without bias: if I can test from a place of complete openness to receive any answer that comes, total acceptance of my not-knowing what the answer should be, then I can get out of my own way enough to receive accurate answers. And if you think about it, that is really the only way I can get accurate answers about my patients. If I have a bias toward a certain answer when I am muscle-testing a patient, if I am prejudiced toward a particular outcome, I am not going to be able to receive information that is clear and true. This open, accepting, receptive state is the state of higher consciousness that Dr. Goswami was referring to when he spoke about connecting with the quantum realm. Goswami called this the state of compassion; he used the term "deep compassion." Valerie Hunt refers to this state - the opening between the human and cosmic mind-fields—as "deep intuition." Barbara Brennan refers to this as love; the energy of the fourth layer of the auric field, the layer related to the heart, "...the transforming crucible through which all energy must pass when going from one world to the other."[35]

Compassion, then, is acceptance of the idea that there is an answer, a reason, for everything; even the things we don't understand, even the things we don't like, even pain. Intuition is the openness to receiving and understanding these higher answers. Neutrality, the optimum state for muscle-testing, for healing work, and most importantly for self-healing, is the level of consciousness that opens us to compassion and intuition. It is a suspension of disbelief that allows for connection with the quantum realm. It is the state of surrender, of trust. It is the state of not-knowing, the state of grace.

CHAPTER 3

WALKING THE PATHWAY

"Great leaps in levels of consciousness are always preceded by surrender of the illusion that 'I know'." [36]

NANCY (the final piece)

I test through a series of energetic points on Nancy, looking for the non-physical sources of her pain, and am shown that the problem is in her nose. Now intellectually, this makes no sense because Nancy didn't have any trauma related to her nose in the car accident. And why, exactly, would her nose cause headaches? Knowing better, at this point, than to question the answers I've been given, I go with it. I ask Nancy to tell me what happened to her nose.

Nancy's next breath comes as a hiss, as if the question literally stings. She hesitates for a long, heavy moment, and then she begins to cry. She cries for a long time, unable to answer my question, unable to stop the flow of tears. It feels like I've tapped into a veritable sea of unshed tears, the force of which, confined in the relatively small area of her nose, has created an unbearable pressure. Hence the headaches. The energy of these tears is potent; as I sit quietly, holding Nancy's head in my hands, I feel their sadness, anger, betrayal, and fear come pouring outward. I feel my own eyes welling up, just from the pure intensity of emotion streaming around me.

Finally, Nancy can speak.

When I was 13 years old, I lived in a small town, in my country, which was very simple and very poor. One day, my father told me that we were going to see a doctor. My mother died when I was very young, so my father was the one who took care of me. We had to ride the bus to the city, which was about an hour away. When we arrived to the doctor's office, I was taken, alone, into a small surgical room where the doctor performed surgery on my nose. Apparently, my father had decided that my nose made me look too Indian, and that if I wanted to find a husband, my nose needed to be smaller. He only explained this to me afterward. The doctor was apparently a friend of my father's, and so he was doing the surgery as a favor. He told me absolutely nothing about what he was going to do to me; he just told me to lie down on the table, he injected me with some type of local anesthetic, and then pulled out the scalpel and started cutting. His one instruction to me was that I must not, under any circumstance, move or cry during the procedure. I was terrified, so of course I obeyed.

I am stunned. Nauseated. I am a chiropractor for many reasons, but one of them is that just the thought of blood and open wounds and exposed bones and such, turns my stomach. I could never be a surgeon. I ask Nancy if she experienced any pain during the surgery.

Not pain, but I could feel the scrape of the knife, and hear the dull tap of the hammer against my face bones. I wanted to scream, or run away, but I couldn't so I just lay there wondering if I was going to die. I didn't move, and I didn't cry.

I relate to Nancy my impression of unshed tears, and all of the trapped and stagnant emotional energy that had been stored up behind her nose. The intense nature of these emotions, and the amount of time they had been festering there, made them very toxic. No wonder she was suffering with headaches. Allowing herself to cry, and to talk about her experience will go a long way toward alleviating the pressure, and relieving the headaches. But I have to wonder, if this horrific experience occurred when Nancy was 13 years old, why she never had headaches until recently—until her car accident?

No Accidents

As trite as this may sound, I don't believe in accidents. Of course the person who rear-ended Nancy didn't do it on purpose, and I'm sure that Nancy didn't plan, much less want, to have an accident. Nonetheless, I think that there is reason for everything. In fact, I think there is good reason for everything. We waste so much of our time and energy in life wondering, "Why me?" This implies that we are the victims of our circumstances, and that there is something wrong with what has happened to us, or worse, that there is just something wrong with *us*. The result is life from the negative perspective. This is one option, and there are essentially two others, as I see it. The second option is the zero perspective: we are not victims, and there is nothing wrong; it's just that "shit happens", as they say. This is certainly a less stressful choice than constant victimhood, but not all that satisfying, you have to admit. The third option is the positive perspective: everything that comes to us is *for* us, according to some benevolent plan, some invisible law of physics that says that everything must grow, must evolve in a direction that is meaningful, purposeful, and inevitably good. Every experience has something to be gleaned from it that will help us evolve. Which of these three options you choose is up to you entirely, since you could argue the validity of all three, but never definitively prove the truth of any one. Except perhaps to yourself.

Working With the Energy

I ask Nancy if there is any situation going on in her life now that is similar in dynamic to her experience as a 13 year old, reminding her of the basic themes behind the emotional energy that was causing her headaches: powerlessness, domination/betrayal by men, inability to move (trapped) or to cry (emotional repression), just to name a few. She nods. I can see the gears whirring in her head for a moment, as a slow smile lights up her face.

It's good to see Nancy smiling.

We talk about her life now. She tells me that her employer is a good man, but he expects more of her than she can give. He wants her to function as a stand-in mother to his son, asking her to live in their home for weeks at a time while he travels on business, frequently (ever so coincidentally) to her native country. When he is gone, she carries all of the responsibility of a mother, but has none of the power; she is expected to care for all of her young charge's needs, but has no authority to make decisions related to those needs. Exhausted and frustrated, but not wanting to upset the little boy, she has been keeping it all to herself. She has thought about looking for another job, but doesn't want to leave the little boy, knowing as she does what it feels like not to have a mother. Of course she hasn't spoken to her employer about the situation, being reluctant to confront him. I think she realizes, as she speaks, how much this has been bothering her.

So she had an accident. Again, I don't actually think she wanted to have an accident, but she really needed to stop and take a good look at the direction she was headed, and choose otherwise. She had herself all tied up in the same situation as her 13 year old self: powerless, unable to move, unable to express herself. And so the persistent headaches. Her higher self gave her a clear, unignorable signal that she needed to address these emotions, and the beliefs that hold them in place: we feel powerless because we believe that others are more powerful than us, we are afraid to move away from, or express dissatisfaction with our circumstances because we believe that it is not safe to do so. Or that we don't deserve to do so. We fear that we are less than, inadequate, wrong in some way.

Oh yeah, that ego thing again.

I ask Nancy to relax and breathe deeply once again. I instruct her to envision the energy that has been trapped in her head moving out with each breath, using the breath as a sort of a pump. As she exhales, the sadness, anger, and fear move out of her body. As she inhales, she draws fresh energy into the same area. I ask her to put her intention into each breath, and draw into her head energy of a higher quality. Think about it: if you evict sadness, anger, and fear, what energy would you want to replace it?

Choose that.

I can feel her whole body smiling now, drawing in the positive energy, and embracing the idea that she can choose her own signature energy. When she's ready, I give her the chiropractic adjustment that she came in for, sure now that it will have an effect.

Nancy comes in again a week later, headache free. She returns for her final evaluation 2 weeks after that, still with no headaches, but with a new job. She is now working as an aide to an elderly woman. The work is much easier, she says, both physically and emotionally. She had a long conversation with her former employer, and then helped him find someone to replace her. She had a long talk with her boy too. They cried together, and then worked out an arrangement where she goes to visit him regularly, but not to work, just to play.

CHAPTER 4

SIGNATURE ENERGY WORK

Your signature energy is a living fabric, woven over the course of many lifetimes; each thread constructed from the feelings that you have experienced over eons of time, and the beliefs that you formulated in response to those feelings. This is the garment that you wear as you move through life in the physical world. As Amit Goswami says, "At one level, we identify with our ego, our story lines. At a deeper level, we realize that we depend on a deeper self, the quantum self, to discover the context of our story lines."[37] In his remarkable book, *Physics of the Soul*, Goswami uses his knowledge of quantum physics, as well as his familiarity with Eastern philosophy and Western psychology, to explain the phenomena of reincarnation by pointing out that the quantum self, being pure energy/information/light, is not subject to the restraints of the ego, to the phenomena of life and death as we normally think of it. Energy cannot be destroyed. Although the individual "story lines", the ego-driven masks that are developed during a particular physical experience (a life) do not continue beyond that life, the themes that underlie the superficial details of our lives, that are formed by the choices that we make from life to life, do continue. In terms of our lamp analogy, when the lamp is old and rusted and no longer functions, we can bring a new lamp home, and plug it in. The wiring, outlets, and even the structure of the house may change, but when we flip the switch, we have light. The human body comes to an end; the human being does not.

The purpose of Signature Energy Work is to consciously explore and understand the history and structure of your signature energy, as a means to improve it. Much of the information is stored beyond the level of consciousness—behind and beyond the walls of the house, so to speak, in the subconscious and superconscious levels—so its influence on you, and on those around you, is not always something that you are aware of. The subconscious mind is devoted to the survival of the individual physical body, so a huge portion of the subconscious energy is based in fear: the fear of death of the physical body. The subconscious is what the ancient Hawaiians called *elemental consciousness*[38], a consciousness that does not rely on reason or logic. It experiences everything literally—only as it occurs, including the thoughts and feelings handed down by the conscious mind. The subconscious mind makes no choices, it merely records the information that is taken in via the physical senses, storing it according to emotional patterns, and handing it back to the conscious mind when called on. Because its job is "creating, re-creating, and maintaining our physical bodies," [39] it never sleeps. Under hypnosis people have recovered memories of events that happened during sleep or surgery, showing that the awareness of the subconscious is always present, always recording and storing information, and always overseeing the involuntary functions that sustain the body toward a singular goal; survival. According to the science of nonlinear dynamics, the more often a particular stimulus is recorded in the subconscious, the larger the probability that we will respond to it in the same way[39]. The denser the subconscious "file" under a particular emotional heading is, the more habitual and ingrained our response patterns will be, so when we respond merely from subconscious patterning, we eliminate choice. We respond by default.

The superconscious mind is the consciousness of the non-physical self, the quantum self. This aspect of our being vibrates at frequencies that are higher than physical form, and is constantly expanding to higher frequencies of vibration. Scientists have demonstrated this expansion and ascension of energy using super-computers and sophisticated mathematics. They developed models for the genesis of our universe from the theoretical "Big Bang"—the explosion of the initial matter of the universe—and found that shortly after the Bang, the force of the explosion had catapulted a full 90% of the matter to vibrational frequencies that are beyond our visible range, in fact beyond our measurable range.[41] To the human perception, 90% of the matter in the universe "disappeared" within seconds after the creation of the universe. Similarly, the superconscious mind, and superconscious memory, are not located in the physical brain, but instead lie in the vibrational range that is beyond our physical perception, in the higher vibrational levels of the human being, the quantum self. Responses to physical stimuli, and events in our lives, can come from the superconscious memory only when our consciousness is focused at these higher frequencies: superconscious responses have to be consciously chosen. As we said earlier (in Chapter 2), the doorway to the superconscious is compassion, the vibrational frequency of unconditional neutrality. Compassion, and most importantly compassion directed toward our own selves, is the impulse that instantly expands and elevates our conscious awareness toward the unlimited enormity of the superconscious. Compassion is the fuel that catapults our consciousness to superconscious levels, that projects our awareness toward the superconscious aspect of our own signature energy. And when we become fully aware of all aspects of our signature energy, we can manage it differently. We can then devote more of our energy to the pursuit and expression of our purpose, which is far beyond mere survival. We become free to contribute our energy toward our aspirations, rather than our fears.

* * * * * * * * *

Becoming aware of the signature energy means becoming conscious of the nature and content of our subconscious files, discarding the files that no longer serve us, and choosing new files that work for us from the repertoire of our superconscious, our quantum self. This clearing and reordering of the signature energy can be a convoluted process that feels a lot like cleaning out your garage: a dusty, sometimes confusing and chaotic uncovering of things you had long forgotten, and often can't remember why in the world you hung on to. The best way to approach it is one step at a time.

CHAPTER 5

STEP ONE: IDENTIFY THE CORE QUESTION

The first step in Signature Energy Work is to identify the core question around which today's session will be centered: what is the problem that needs to be solved, or the understanding that is to be gained at this time? What is the thread in the signature energy garment that is ready to be rewoven or replaced today? Or, what's on top of the pile in *your* garage? Because I am a chiropractor, many of my patients' presenting problems are pain. Again, I look at pain as the body's way of trying to get our attention, in effect saying to us, "Start here! Please!" The question I ask, then, is about the pain: specifically, the cause of the pain. I can ask my patient where his pain is, but I may have to ask his quantum self where the source of this pain is, and more importantly, what the purpose of the pain is.

Let me interject here with the stipulation that Signature Energy Work is *not* meant to be a substitute for medical care. If I have a patient who comes to me with a physical complaint, it is my duty to rule out an urgent medical problem, and to treat or refer the patient for treatment that is appropriate. Signature Energy Work may be an appropriate treatment in this situation, it just may not be the only treatment needed, and if there is a medical emergency, not the first treatment that should be given. When pain is involved, Signature Energy Work is most appropriately used on chronic pain, or pain that has not resolved with mainstream medical care. This statement can also be applied to non-physical pain, which is another reason that people seek Signature Energy Work. I am referring to emotional pain; when there is nothing physically wrong with you, you don't hurt anywhere, but you just *feel* bad.

Signature energy work can be very helpful here, of course, but once again the presence of serious illness, in this case psychological or psychiatric in nature, should first be ruled out.

Often patients come to me because their primary forms of healthcare are not quite solving their problem, or they just feel the need to understand their life experience better. They want to know *why*? Why am I having this experience? This illness, this pain, this problem? And why *now*? What does it mean? They may not have any idea what "energy-work" is, but if they are curious enough to ask these questions, they are ready for Signature Energy Work. Sam is a perfect example of this.

CASE STUDY #2 – SAM

Sam had been coming to my office for years. He came only occasionally at first, and then only on the insistence of his wife. He was extremely skeptical of any type of alternative medicine, having come from a traditional medical background; his father had been a medical doctor in the small town where Sam grew up. Sam spent many hours as a child watching sick people going in to his father's home-office, and coming out again after receiving an injection or precisely-worded prescription, or, if the case was bad, a ride in an ambulance to the hospital in the larger town nearby. This was Sam's familiar concept of medicine.

Sam often complained of stiffness in his mid-back, and came to me strictly for chiropractic adjustments to this area—and then only because it gave him immediate, albeit temporary, relief. Over time, he also mentioned to me that he suffered with frequent episodes of gastric bloating and a sense of heaviness around the liver. When he was very stressed, he would develop small ulcers in his mouth, on the tongue and insides of his lips. His wife spoke to him repeatedly, and enthusiastically, about her experiences with Signature Energy Work. He mentioned this to me while in my office one day, and asked if I could "tell him some things about himself".

His physical complaint on that day was the usual one, general stiffness and sudden acute mid-back spasms. I asked him to lie face-down on my table, so that I could examine the mid-back area and do some deep massage work there first, mostly as a way to let him know that I was aware of the extent of his physical pain, and to "loosen up" his energy. As I worked on some of the rock-hard muscular knots in his thoracic paraspinal muscles, I explained that this particular area of the spine is where the nerves that feed the liver, gallbladder, and stomach have their roots, and suggested that his back pain may be related to his digestive symptoms. I told him that it was possible for one to be causing the other, but more likely they were both just symptoms of the same problem. It would be interesting to know where that problem was coming from. He asked if I could find out, and said that he would really like to understand why he had digestive problems, since his doctors could never find anything "wrong" with him. With this, I knew Sam was finally ready for some Signature Energy Work.

Preparation

The readiness of a person to participate in Signature Energy Work is often reflected in the words that the patient uses to describe his complaints. I listen to his words, and the emotional charge behind them, to find out what his problem means to him: what he wants, and is willing, to change. Sometimes—often actually—the patient doesn't really want to change, he just wants things to be different. (This, some say, is the definition of insanity; at the philosophical level, if not the clinical.) He wants his *problem* to change without *him* having to change. He wants someone else to fix it. In our modern society, this is normal; it's the way that most of us were raised. We go to the doctor; the doctor cures us. Our job is to be a good patient, to be passive and cooperative. Compliant. It can be a long walk from compliant to curious. Signature Energy Work often starts with teaching my patient why he might want to participate in *understanding* his problem. This means cultivating in him the realization that his problem has a reason behind it, and that understanding this reason is not only the first step toward creating a solution, but also an avenue for self-exploration and growth. This realization is a process: a process of learning about the multi-dimensional nature of our own energy, about the power of self-awareness, about personal freedom and personal responsibility. Any process takes time, and has specific steps toward its endpoint. The words a person chooses, the tone and the body language that back them up, inform me about where he is in that process: how committed he is to changing, and where his understanding and beliefs are about change. This is a vital indicator of where our session needs to start, and how fast we should proceed. Often, as with Sam, it's necessary to start slowly, creating rapport and feeding the patient little bytes of spiritual and energetic concepts – how they create their physical reality from their consciousness, how their emotional, mental, and spiritual bodies affect their physical body—weaning them off of their medical passivity, until they reach the point where a more active level of Signature Energy Work is indicated.

    It also happens that patients show up quite ready for, and open to energy-work, but are so enmeshed with physical pains and personal issues that they have no idea where to start. Listening is key here. It is important for the patient to have an opportunity to talk, to give their version of what is happening to them, but in addition, listening to a patient's history often provides me with clues as to the nature of the patient's core question. Patients may touch on several different types of problems that they are experiencing, physically and/or emotionally, and there is usually a common theme among them. Within the common theme usually lies the single, pressing question whose answer would catalyze great change for the patient.

Let me use my patient Margaret as an example.

CASE STUDY #3 – MARGARET

Margaret is a successful professional woman who is approaching 50. She came to me on this particular day complaining of lower back pain and fatigue, which she related to her chronic problems with uterine fibroid tumors. She spoke briefly about her mother, whose care Margaret had been overseeing for the past 7 years since being diagnosed with Alzheimer's disease. We had worked together on Margaret's mother issues, and their relation to her fibroids, many times, from many angles. Margaret had progressed beautifully on the subject, experiencing incredible growth and expansion in her life as a result. But Margaret had also long been feeling the financial and emotional strain of her mother's illness, on both herself and her family, and wondered why her mother just seemed to hang on to life, in spite of being completely removed from it mentally. Margaret went on to talk about her work, her stresses and her ambitions there, and made particular mention of her co-worker, Jill, who appeared to be dealing with terminal cancer. (Margaret knew that Jill had cancer, but was unable to obtain a lot of details from Jill about her illness.) In spite of her obvious health problems, Jill was still coming to work each day and performing her duties in her usual cold, distant, but highly professional manner. While feeling a deep sadness and compassion for Jill, and sympathizing with her apparent reluctance to let anyone help her, for fear they might pity her, Margaret had noticed that Jill had taken to following her almost everywhere she went in the office. Margaret's job required her to handle several different projects at one time, which resulted in her moving from one station to another quite frequently. It seemed that wherever Margaret went within the office over the course of the day, Jill would inevitably find a way to put herself there also. Jill's nearly unfillable need to be in Margaret's presence throughout the workday was becoming quite draining for Margaret. She didn't want to be unkind, but she just couldn't see what Jill needed that she, Margaret, could offer. I was struck by the remarkable parallel between Margaret's situation with her mother and with Jill. I suggested that we muscle test Margaret on the core question, "What is available for Margaret to learn in her relation with Jill?" knowing that this would probably help Margaret see what was still available for her to learn in her relation with her mother. Margaret responded with that wide-eyed, slow nod of the head that tells me I've hit the target: a question that sends the brain into overdrive, that no logic or reasoning can answer satisfactorily.

A question for the quantum realm.

Focus

While listening to my patient is important, some patients just don't like to talk. Because I am a chiropractor, people tend to approach me according to their preconceived definition of chiropractic medicine: they think they should only talk about their physical pain, and its physical causes. It doesn't occur to them to address the non-physical in a chiropractor's office. They essentially just point to where it hurts, and then lie down on my table and wait for me to "fix" them. In addition, there are many patients who haven't developed the self-awareness to notice the link between their thoughts and emotions and their physical pain, and even some who are so accustomed to tuning out their pain, perhaps because they are too busy to stop and acknowledge it, that they aren't fully aware of where their physical pain is located.

They know that their back hurts, but they may not really know what I can do about it. They came to see me only because their friend, or therapist, or even their doctor told them to give me a call. These people come to get fixed without having any clear idea what's broken. I confess that I still have a very difficult time mastering my enthusiasm (and my heroic aspirations) in this situation; after all, I have so much more to offer a patient than just "fixing their back!" But in these cases, we can skirt both the patient's limited beliefs and my own ego by focusing on a more generic core question, "What do we need to work on today?" Maybe all we need to work on *is* their back, but the quantum realm frequently presents us with much more interesting things. As with Miranda, for example.

CASE STUDY #4 – MIRANDA

Miranda is a woman in her 50's, who looks much younger due to her beautiful blond, athletic physique. She is fiercely active and impeccably fit. Her Pilates instructor referred her to me, thinking that Miranda might have some non-physical "issues" that were holding up her progress in class. When I asked Miranda what she wanted to work on in our session, she spoke at length: about old injuries that she had suffered that resulted in occasional stiffness in various areas of her body, about being at an age where it seemed important to involve herself in a process of transformation in order to move forward in her life, about freeing herself from past patterns, about committing herself to personal growth. In other words, she had no idea. This gave me the general impression that she was open to Signature Energy Work, but didn't give me much to go on as to the nature of the core question for our session. So, I had her lie on the table, and muscle tested the question, "Is there a particular issue that we need to work on today?"

Yes.

OK, good. I proceeded to muscle test through my SEWLINE questions (see Chapter 6) until I arrived at the conclusion that the core problem to be worked on that day involved releasing energy from Miranda's heart chakra; specifically, an energy related to her husband. This information gave me a focus for the treatment, but it also presented an opportunity for Miranda to examine the energies in her heart chakra—she apparently had some garage-cleaning to do there.

(This illustrates my point about framing a core question for the session, but I'm going to stretch your attention a bit in order to finish Miranda's story now; it's a good story, and it proves my point about having more interesting things to work on.)

I put my hand gently over Miranda's sternum, and said, "We're going to move some energy in your heart chakra today," at which point she sighed deeply, and closed her eyes. I explained that the energy to be moved was energy that she had been holding on to, and that was ready to be released. And, I added, she was ready to release it. In fact, I told her, she had probably been sent to me at this time, on this day, *because* she was ready to release it, and just needed me to tell her so. I went on to explain that this energy belonged to her husband: specifically, her husband at 36 years of age. I asked Katherine what happened to her husband when he was 36. She answered briskly,

"That's when his son died."

Ouch. She answered so quickly, and so matter-of-factly, that I almost missed the importance of what she said. But when I turned my attention from her heart chakra (where I was feeling a deep ache pushing against my hands), to her face, I couldn't miss the tightening of her jaw against the slow trail of a tear down her cheek.

She explained that she had known her husband when he was 36, but she was not married to him then. Nonetheless, I explained, she seemed to be holding her husband's unprocessed energy about losing his son in her heart chakra, probably as a way of helping him deal with it. It was time for her to find a way to give it back to him.

Long pause. She said she had no idea how to do that. Her body language said she really, really wanted to, but wouldn't if it meant hurting her husband.

So Miranda was trapped between helping herself and hurting her husband. A familiar stance for those of us learning the delicate art of love and compassion, I think.

I asked her to first take a few deep breaths, then to look at the inside of her heart, in whatever way she knew how to do that, in order to see the energy that was there—the energy that was her husband's. She blinked a few times, breathed deeply, visibly relaxed her body, then nodded. She was there. Next I instructed her to ask the energy, in whatever way it seemed appropriate to her to ask, how she could best go about giving the energy back to her husband.

She was quiet for a few moments, and then said,

"Through his poetry. Collaborate with him, listen to him through the words of his poetry."

Miranda explained that she and her husband were leaving the next day to spend the summer traveling in Europe. They would have lots of quality alone-time in which to share ideas, and feelings, around his poetry. This meant that she would have to finish the treatment over the course of the summer, without any supervision from me. She would have to trust her instincts about it, but I was confident that she could. (And besides, I'm sorry, but it's just impossible to worry about a woman who is traveling through

Europe with a man who writes poetry...) And he would have plenty of time to write while they were away. Perfect opportunity, perfect timing.

Once again I asked Miranda to look into her heart chakra, but this time to examine her own inherent energy there. What was the quality of her own heart chakra energy that resonated with her husband's loss and grief for his son, that had in fact attracted his energy to take up residence in her heart chakra?

More tears, this time not so controlled, and from a much deeper place.

"For the past 7 years, I've been separated from my own sons."

The terms of their divorce agreement were such that Miranda's first husband kept their two boys living with him until they finished high-school. She had spent the last 7 years watching them grow up from a distance, and the thought crossed my mind that this distance must have felt like the same eternity to her as her current husband's separation from his son felt like to him. Every day felt like a lifetime.

But Miranda's boys had come back to her. Her oldest was now in college, and her youngest just graduating high school, and preparing to come live with her full-time.

Then I asked the hard question: what good had come from the separation? What was she able to see, right now, that only the experience of separation could have shown her? What had she learned from it, that she probably wouldn't have any other way? And what about her boys: how had they grown from the experience?

She realized there were many ways that they had all grown, from the fundamental and profound, to the minute and even amusing. Miranda's tears were bitter-sweet now. Perhaps she could

SIGNATURE ENERGY WORK

help her husband see that some good had, or at least could, come from his separation from his son. And perhaps open him to the possibility that their separation too was, ultimately, only temporary.

Find the Core

It may takes months, even years, for a patient to be ready for the level of self-exploration involved in Signature Energy Work. And it may take careful intuitive listening, or slow and patient searching to find the core question for muscle-testing. But occasionally I get a patient who is so obviously ready for Signature Energy Work that very little preparation or explanation is necessary. Then I can head straight to the point, saying simply, "If you could ask the universe any question, and get an answer, what question would you want to ask?"

CASE STUDY #5 - MARIA

Maria cried when I asked her that question.

"*I just want to know why...why does this keep happening to me?*"

Maria was referred to my office by her friend, a patient of mine, who told Maria that I could treat her occasional lower back pain using traditional chiropractic medicine, but also encouraged her to ask me about Signature Energy Work. By the time Maria made an appointment with me, she was not actually having any back pain, but the idea of energy-work was intriguing to her. She explained that she is an artist, a dancer, and that in spite of her training, experience, skill, and talent, she always seemed to be out of work. Struggling to keep up with her most basic living expenses, she was becoming tired, hopeless, and depressed. A few years back she made the decision to quit her "day job" in favor of devoting herself to what she considered her real work, dance. She had performed in dozens of dance jobs that looked like tremendous opportunities initially, but always seemed to turn into dead-ends where she had to fight to get paid, the show was canceled, or she was unappreciated or misunderstood in some way. The friend who referred her to me had indeed mentioned Maria's enormous talent, and confirmed that Maria never seemed to get a break in the dance world. The thought of going back to work in a 9-to-5 job would be considered complete failure by Maria, who felt very strongly that dance was her gift, and that she was meant to share it.

She never felt depressed when she was on-stage. She felt the joy of touching her audience, of sweeping them up into her tremendous passion for the beauty of the dance. Within minutes of leaving the stage, however, the darkness would begin to return. She had noticed a few months prior that this was often accompanied by feeling as if her heart was beating too fast. This scared her enough to pay a visit to her medical doctor, who ran a series of tests, determined that there was "nothing wrong with her," and prescribed an anti-depressant medication. Maria discontinued the medication after a few weeks, unable to tolerate how it made her feel. She had tried several forms of psycho-therapy, massage, acupuncture and even energetic healing and spiritual counseling, but had not experienced any significant change in her condition, or her situation. She really needed an answer.

* * * * * * * * *

Once I have established the core question for which the patient is seeking an answer, I can turn to muscle-testing to begin the search. Very often I find myself centering my muscle testing around some form of the question, "Why?" Why does Nancy have headaches? Why does Maria have such a problem succeeding at her work? If you recall, however, with muscle-testing the questions must be asked in a yes-or-no format. In Nancy's case it might have taken me years to go from "Why does Nancy have headaches?" to, "Is the problem located in Nancy's nose?" What's needed is a simple path that will take us from a "why" question to a "yes" (or "no") answer.

    I am, by nature, a simplifier. In over 20 years of clinical experience, I have come across many muscle-testing systems, and "protocols" for asking questions through muscle-testing, in many different contexts. I tend to glean what I like best from a complex protocol, and then simplify to suit my own needs. I have integrated each system with my own healing experiences and philosophies, to create a system that works for me. The result is a comfortably simple, but reasonably comprehensive line of questions that I call the SEW (Signature Energy Work) LINE (of questioning). This book is meant to be a teaching tool for you to learn my system, but I am obviously not a purist, so I encourage you to examine my SEWLINE, understand it, master it, and then use it as a starting point. Examine your own healing background, beliefs, and interests, and then create your own line of questions. Use it for your own self-exploration and healing. Apply it to your already existing healing practice, be it personal or professional.

    As I stated in the Introduction, I believe that healing is an art. When you master the technical structure of any healing modality or system, you become a technician, but when you stand on that structure and leap from it into the unknown, you become an artist.

CHAPTER 6

STEP TWO: FIND THE ANSWER

The SEWLINE is a method for analyzing your personal energy field—your signature energy (or the signature energy of your patient)—in order to find an answer to the core question. As I stated in the earlier chapters, energy is essentially made up of tiny particles of light/information that function together as a field, and travel in waves. Each human energy field has unique qualities associated with it; some of those qualities are measurable by traditional objective means, and some qualities can only be perceived subjectively. The same is true for the energy field associated with inanimate objects, like a planet or a weather system, or for the energy field of less tangible things, like a thought or a feeling. The signature energy of the answer to our core question—the *core answer*—is therefore made up of tiny particles of information, which come together to form an energetic field possessing unique qualities; qualities which, when perceived by us, reveal its nature. The more detailed an understanding we have of the nature of the energy of our core answer, the clearer that answer will be for us. The SEWLINE is a system for examining, in detail, the energetic qualities of the core answer.

The specific qualities of energy that I find most helpful (and interesting) to study are listed in Diagram A.

SIGNATURE ENERGY WORK

LOCATION
    Levels of the Field
    Chakras
    Organs
    Body Regions
DIRECTION
    In
    Out
BLOCK
    Entry
    Exit
THE SIX W'S
    Who
    What
    When
    Where
    How
    Why

(Diagram A – SEWLINE)

Levels of the Field
    All levels
    Physical level
    Emotional level
    Mental level
    Spiritual level

Chakras
    1st through 7th
    8th through 12th

Organs
    Lungs
    Heart
    Liver
    Gallbladder
    Stomach
    Pancreas
    Spleen
    Small Intestine
    Kidneys
    Adrenal Glands
    Large Intestine
    Sexual/Reproductive Organs
    Urinary Bladder

Body Regions
    Upper Extremities
    Lower Extremities
    Head and neck
    Back
    Chest
    Abdomen
    Hara

Specific Structures

(Diagram B – LOCATION)

LOCATION

The first quality of energy that I examine with the SEWLINE is "location." What is the location, within our personal signature energy field, of the signature energy field of our core answer? And what does the nature of that location tell me about the nature of the core answer? Where, in the energetic garment that is my (or my patient's) signature energy, is the thread that relates to this core question, and it's answer? Where, in our energetic home, does the change need to be made, if we flip the lightswitch and the lamp does not go on? It may not help to just replace the lightbulb. What if the lamp is not plugged in, or we haven't paid the electric bill? If we establish where the problem is actually occurring—from lamp, to wiring, to transformers, to power plant—we can make the appropriate "adjustment", or do the appropriate "work," to solve the problem.

Levels of the Field

In searching for a location, I want to start from the broadest perspective first, and then gradually narrow my focus, so I begin my SEWLINE questions from the perspective of the layers, or levels of the energy field.

In my searching I have found dozens of descriptions, from hundreds of sources—ancient cultures to modern science—for the levels of the human energy field; and while these descriptions differ, the similarities between them are startling. In the Upanishads, the ancient scriptures forming the last portion of the Hindu *Vedas*, the human energy field is described as consisting of five "bodies". The first is the gross physical body, called *annamaya*. The next, more "subtle", or less dense body is called *pranamaya,* because it is thought to be made of *prana,* or vital energy. The next, even subtler body is called *manomaya*, made of *mana,* or mind substance. Next is the *vijnanamaya*, made of *vijnana,* or supramental intelligence; this is referred to as the theme body, because it is thought to hold the context for the lower three bodies. (In other words, the content of the lower three bodies exists within the unifying structure of the theme body. The *content* of our "lower bodies" – our physical appearance, emotional reactions, and superficial thought processes – changes from lifetime to lifetime, but the *structure* of our "lower bodies" - the overarching theme - is contiguous. The furnishings and décor in our energetic home change, but the structure of the house stays the same.) Last is the *anandamaya*, made of the most subtle of all energies, *ananda,* or spiritual bliss; this is referred to as the bliss body, or Brahman – the ground of all being. Each subtle body is said to extend progressively farther from the gross physical body, with the bliss body being limitless in its scope.

Compare this description of the human energy field from the Upanishads with that from the Kabbalah, the ancient teachings of Jewish mysticism, where again we find five layers. The Kabbalah discusses five "worlds", with five corresponding subtle bodies. First is the ground of being, called the *Ain Sof,* the divine manifestation of the one into many. The Ain Sof manifests itself through the *Atziluth*, the world of pure thought (archetypes and themes); *Briah*, the world that puts meaning to creation (thoughts and emotions); *Yetzirah*, the world of morphogenesis (the energetic blueprint for biological form); and *Assiah*, the physical manifestation of form (the gross physical world). Both of these systems fit with the observations of Barbara Brennan, as noted in Chapter 1, of etheric physical, emotional, mental, and spiritual layers of the human energy field, all surrounding the gross physical body. I also mentioned previously the system of the ancient Hawaiians, the Huna concepts. The Huna saw the human being as consisting of three "selves," functioning in three different levels of consciousness.[42] The three selves were known as the lower self, middle self, and High Self; or *unihipili, uhane,* and *Aumakua.* The lower self was said to live in the realm of nature; of biological intelligence, or "elemental" consciousness, which is the intelligence thought to be in all animated physical bodies. The middle self is in the realm of human consciousness, our social consciousness. The Higher Self is at the level of divine consciousness. Interestingly, in the Hawaiian language, all three selves are referred to as "spirits," implying that all of the three selves are beyond the gross physical form. A nature spirit is said to control the physical body, a human spirit resides temporarily in the body as a guest of the nature spirit, and surrounding the physical body is the divine spirit. While these three "selves" closely mirror the three levels of consciousness found in modern Western psychology, I am struck by the similarity of the "lower self" of the Huna, to the "lower bodies" of the Upanishads. Equally striking is the parallel between the "middle self" of the Huna, the *vijnanamaya* of the Upanishads, and the *Atziluth* of the Kaballah; perhaps implying that the human spirit is actually of "supramental" consciousness—relating to the themes and archetypes that have no physical form, and which transcend time. In Christian mysticism this middle self, the supramental human spirit, is called the soul.[43] If you recall, Barbara Brennan referred to the middle "layer" of the human energy field as that which relates to the heart, and the energy of love.

(Which perhaps suggests that what draws the human soul to take residence in the human body is love; the opportunity to experience love through the format of physicality. That would be the subject for a very long, if very interesting, discussion...)

These levels of the human energy field also remind me of the evolutionary levels of structure and function of the human brain, which I studied so long ago in chiropractic college. I was blessed with a very diligent and passionate neuroanatomy professor (whose name I have long ago forgotten—thank-you sir, wherever you are now), who made us learn, understand, and memorize every nook and cranny of the human brain, presented as a four-fold system. The oldest part of this system is the hindbrain, often referred to as our reptilian brain, because it is the same brain that is found in reptilian species. It consists of our sensory motor system – the spinal cord and its vast network of nerves throughout the body – and its function is to handle the survival of the physical body. The next oldest part of the brain is the limbic system, also called the old mammalian brain, as it is the level of brain development found in ancient mammal species. The functions of the limbic system are to add the senses of smell and hearing to our sensory repertoire, and to handle all forms of relationship, from our general cognition that we are separate from the world, and therefore must relate to it as something "other" than ourselves, to our relationships with other living creatures. In other words, the limbic system is in charge of the tool that we use to evaluate all our relationships—our emotions. The third part of the human brain is the neocortex, which introduces language and objective thinking. This is often called the new mammalian brain. You can see the parallels between these three brain systems and the physical, emotional, and mental levels of the human energy field; or with the "lower" self, as described above.

Neuroscientist Paul MacLean, former head of the Department of Brain Evolution and Behavior at the National Institutes of Health, considered the fourth part of the human brain, the prefrontal lobes, to be in charge of our "higher human virtues" of compassion, empathy, and love, as well as our higher intellectual skills, such as our ability to reason, analyze, and think creatively. The prefrontal lobes are the most recent addition to the evolution of the human brain, and they connect to all three of the other parts, through an elaborate network of neural tissues, in order to integrate and regulate our thoughts and emotions. In addition, researchers in the relatively new scientific field of neuro-cardiology have found that the prefrontal lobes connect to a recently discovered brain center located in the human heart.[44] This fact seems to reinforce the concept of a "supramental" level, or "middle" self, one that relates directly to the energies and functions of the heart.

I have found it most practical to work with four basic levels of the signature energy field: the physical level, which includes the gross physical as well as the physical etheric bodies; the emotional level; the mental level, which relates to the "lower" mental energy of our thoughts and cognitive processes; and the spiritual level, which involves the supramental, as well as divine aspects.

To determine which level of the signature energy field is related to our core answer, I muscle test this question:

IS (the answer) RELATED TO A PARTICULAR LEVEL (OR LEVELS) OF THE FIELD?

If the answer to this question is no, then I can assume that the answer relates to all levels of the field.

If this question tests yes, then I test all of the following four questions.

IS IT RELATED TO THE PHYSICAL LEVEL OF THE FIELD?

IS IT RELATED TO THE EMOTIONAL LEVEL?

TO THE MENTAL LEVEL?

TO THE SPIRITUAL LEVEL?

DR. CORA B. LLERA, D.C.

I note the answer to all four questions, because the answer may relate to more than one level. In the case of Nancy, her headaches were related to both the emotional and mental levels, meaning that she had both emotions and thoughts/beliefs that were triggering her headaches. Each level of the field is actually a higher vibrational version of the gross physical body, so we are using the landmarks on the physical body to determine the exact location of the core answer on the non-physical levels. Think of it this way: the human being is like a set of stacking Russian dolls. When you look at the outermost doll, it appears whole and complete. When you pull it open, however, you find another doll, an exact replica only smaller, contained within. You can open up the smaller replica, and again find another exact copy contained within. The human energy field "doll", for purposes of this discussion, contains three more dolls within it. The spiritual doll is largest (limitless, in fact), and contains the mental, emotional, and physical dolls. Any specific location on any level of the field has a corresponding location on all other levels of the field. The location of the nose, for example, on the physical level—the innermost doll—has a corresponding nose on the emotional, mental and spiritual dolls. Nancy, then, had her core problem located in the emotional nose as well as the mental nose: the same location, but on two levels of her field.

It sometimes happens that the patient is not ready, for his own reasons, to address all levels of the signature energy field related to his problem. As a chiropractor, I frequently have patients come to me strictly to work on the physical level, usually because their belief systems don't allow them to venture beyond this level, but occasionally because they are working on the other levels of the field with another type of practitioner (a psychotherapist, for example). In these cases, it is not appropriate (or not necessary) for me to work on all of the levels of the field. Even though it may be apparent to me that other levels are involved with the problem, I work only on the levels that test positive on that day

Chakras

The next focus in my location search is the chakras. The term chakra is becoming more common in our modern culture thanks to the current popularity of yoga. The esoteric and alternative medicine literature is full of descriptions and definitions of the chakras, and every definition that I come upon seems to be slightly different. To make sure we're all on the same page, let me briefly explain my working definition of the term "chakra".

A chakra is a portal, a connecting point of entry between the energetic bodies and the physical body. To use the lamp analogy yet again, the chakras are like dimmer switches. They connect the lamp to the wiring in the walls of our signature energy "home," and regulate how much power comes through to the lamp. Dimmer switch turned up fully—bright light. Dimmer switch turned down low—dim light.

There are references to as many as twelve major chakras in the esoteric literature, but chakras one through seven are the most commonly accepted, and most thoroughly understood. I find myself led most frequently to these "lower" seven, although I have, on occasion, found myself called on to venture into the eighth and ninth chakras also. There is relatively little information available regarding the exact nature and function of the higher chakras, although we can say that they generally relate to our spiritual and divine aspects. I will leave you to research the higher chakras on your own, and for the purposes of this book focus on the first seven, each of which has a specific location on the physical body, with a corresponding gland in that area that is the primary physical manifestation of the energy of that chakra. The chakra acts as a modulator for the energy coming into its area of the body, and, in addition, each chakra modulates a particular type of energy for the entire body. If our core answer is located in a particular chakra, the characteristics of that chakra may give us clues about the characteristics of our answer.

The first chakra is located at the base of the spine, in the area of the coccyx, and is often called the base, or root chakra. This chakra relates to the physical structures of the spine and coccyx, the legs and feet, and certain aspects of the adrenal glands and kidneys. The function of this chakra is to support all of the other chakras, and guard the survival of the physical body by integrating the neural and endocrine systems. The first chakra is associated with physical energy, and processes energies that relate to physical survival and security; most particularly survival and security strategies and issues inherited from our families, our cultural environment, and our past lives.

The second chakra is located at approximately the base of the sacrum, midway between the navel and the pubic bone, and so is often referred to as the sacral chakra. This chakra relates to the physical structure of the reproductive organs, and its function is to guarantee the perpetuation of the human species. It is associated with emotional energy, and processes energies that relate to sexuality, nurturing, and creativity.

The third chakra is located at the center of the diaphragm, approximately the same location as the bundle of nerves called the solar plexus; thus this chakra is often referred to as the solar plexus chakra. It relates to the physical structures of the diaphragm, abdomen, and the abdominal organs, including the liver, gallbladder, stomach and intestines, pancreas and spleen (although some functions of the spleen also relate to the second chakra, and some esoteric texts view the spleen as an additional chakra unto itself). This chakra is associated with mental energy, and its function is to process energies related to our concept of personal power (and its opposite, powerlessness).

The fourth chakra, or heart chakra, is located at the center of the sternum. This chakra relates to the physical structures of the chest and arms, heart, lungs, and thymus gland. Its function is to act as an interface between our lower, physically oriented self, and our higher, spiritually oriented self. It processes energies related to loving and being loved.

The fifth chakra, or throat chakra, is located in the center of the throat, and is associated with the physical structures of the neck, throat, mouth, ears, and thyroid and parathyroid glands. Its function is to channel the higher creative and emotional energies, and blend them with our individual creative energy. This chakra processes issues relating to our self expression.

The sixth chakra is located between the eyebrows, and so is often referred to as the third eye chakra. It relates to the physical structures of the eyes, nose, and the pituitary gland. Ancient esoteric teachers considered this chakra to be the center of the integrated personality, and as such its function is to channel the higher mental energies. Through this chakra we process the energies of imagination and our sense of purpose.

The seventh chakra is located at the top of the head, and is also known as the crown chakra. It relates to the physical structure of the pineal gland, and its function is to act as a channel for higher spiritual energy. Through this chakra we process issues of our relation with, and understanding of, the divine.

To determine whether the core answer is located in a chakra, I muscle test this question:

IS (the answer) LOCATED IN THE CHAKRAS?

If this tests "no", then I can move on to the next question.

If the muscle tests "yes" to this, then I find out more specifically which chakra by asking:

IS (the answer) LOCATED IN CHAKRAS 1-7?

If yes, then I like to locate the specific chakra by holding my hand a few inches above the body, over each chakra, asking "Is this the chakra involved?" and muscle testing. I continue until I find the chakra that tests "yes". I could also just name each chakra, and then test. In the case of my patient Maria, the dancer, the heart chakra tested positive, indicating that the answer to her question (Why does this keep happening to me?) was related to the heart chakra, which made perfect sense in light of her physical symptom of tachycardia.

If the muscle tests "no" to chakras 1-7, then I ask about chakras 8-12:

IS (the answer) LOCATED IN CHAKRAS 8-12?

Organs

The next category of focus for my location search is the organs. Each organ in our body has an anatomical location as well as a specific physiological function. The energetic signature of the organ is a reflection of both its location and its physiology. If the core answer that I am seeking is found in an organ, I use this as an indication of both the location of our answer, and the nature of its energetic signature. A brief explanation of the characteristics of some of the major organs follows.

LUNGS: Lungs regulate the flow of one of our most basic energies, oxygen, into and out of our bodies. Without oxygen, the body cannot sustain life. The lungs process energies and issues related to grief and loss, as well as our sense of being able to "breathe freely."

HEART: The heart, as an organ, is the center point for the flow of blood to the body.
Energetically, the heart is also our center. It processes the energies and issues related to our sense of ourselves as the center of our universe, and our ability and desire to reach outward from that center to connect with the world around us.

LIVER: The liver acts as a filter for toxins in the blood, and produces the bile (also known as gall) that is stored in the gallbladder, and used by the digestive system to break down our food. Energetically, the liver acts as a filter for toxic energy coming to us from our environment, and so processes issues relating to anger. It is also the source of the gall—decisiveness, *chutzpah*—that we use to respond to our environment, and to move forward toward filling our potential.

GALLBLADDER: The gallbladder is a sac, a storage vessel for the fluids and energies of the liver. When the gallbladder is overloaded or congested, the result is a precipitation of the gall into gallstones. Energetically, when the flow of our gall, our ability to move through boundaries and break down obstacles, is bound up, the result is frustration.

STOMACH: The stomach is the beginning of the digestive system, where the food that we eat begins to change into fuel for our body. Energetically, the stomach processes the energies and issues related to our desire for, and ability to process, change.

PANCREAS: The pancreas is the organ that secretes insulin, the hormone that our body uses to process and regulate sugar. Energetically, the pancreas regulates energies and issues involving our sense of "sweetness"—nourishment, pleasure—in our life.

SPLEEN: The spleen is responsible for the production of our lymph and blood cells, which it supplies, in the right amount and at the right time, to the rest of our body in order to replace damaged cells or rebuff invading organisms. Energetically, the spleen processes the energies of worry and rumination, as well as issues relating to empathy and our sense of personal boundaries.

SMALL INTESTINE: The small intestine is the site of digestion, where our food is broken down into its smallest usable elements. Energetically, the small intestine processes energies and issues about our ability to use or understand what's coming at us from our environment.

KIDNEYS: The kidneys act as filters for the blood, and produce urine as a method of disposing of fluid waste products from the blood. The kidneys filter our energetic fluids, our emotions, and process our most fundamental emotion, fear.

ADRENAL GLANDS: The adrenal glands are located directly on top of the kidneys, and secrete hormones that regulate our "fight, flight, or freeze" response to stressors in our environment. In short, the adrenal glands process the energies and issues related to stress. I consider two different types of stress when assessing the adrenal glands: First is what I call "horizontal stress"—the stress that we feel from the ordinary things in our environment; traffic, taxes, and the general sense that we have too much to do, and not enough time to do it. Second is what I call "vertical stress"—our sense of alignment with our place on the Earth, our path or direction in life, as well as our sense of alignment with our Higher Self, our purpose and meaning in life. If the adrenal glands test positive, I like to ask whether horizontal or vertical stress is involved.

LARGE INTESTINE: The large intestine is generally charged with the job of absorbing nutrients from our food, and storing and releasing the leftover unusable waste products. The large intestine is broken into three parts: the ascending colon, transverse colon, and descending colon. The ascending colon functions primarily to absorb the nutritious elements that have been broken down in the small intestine. Energetically, the ascending colon represents our ability to glean the good from our experiences. The transverse colon functions as the transitional level between absorbing nutrients, and sorting out the unusable wastes in preparation for disposal. This represents our ability to transform experience into wisdom, and our ability to know what to keep, and what to let go. The descending colon is the final stop before the evacuation chamber (the rectum), and as such it represents our ability to let go of that which is no longer usable.

SEXUAL/REPRODUCTIVE ORGANS: These organs function in the human body as a mechanism for procreation, as well as for the regulation of our sexual characteristics and functions. Energetically, these organs process the energies and issues involved with sexuality, gender roles, and our sense of physical pleasure.

URINARY BLADDER: The urinary bladder is the vessel that holds the fluids filtered from the blood by the kidneys. The bladder is responsible for holding these fluids until such time as release is appropriate. Energetically, the bladder processes the fluid energies – emotions – that are no longer relevant, and need to be released.

To determine whether the core answer is located in an organ, I muscle test this question:

IS (the answer) LOCATED IN THE ORGANS?

If "yes", then I find which organ is specifically involved by placing my hand on the patient's body, over the location of each of the main organs one at a time, testing each organ in the same fashion as the chakras described above.

If organs test "no", then I go on to the next question.

Body Regions

Each region of the body has a general location and physiologic function, as well as a general energetic pattern. To find whether the core answer is located in a body region, I muscle test this question:

IS (answer) LOCATED IN A PARTICULAR BODY REGION?

If "yes", I test each region individually until I find the region that tests "yes".

UPPER EXTREMITIES: In general the upper extremities (which include the arms and hands) are used to reach out toward the world around us, or to hold the world away from us. Energetically, they function as accessories to the heart chakra.

LOWER EXTREMITIES: The lower extremities (which include the legs and feet) are what connect our bodies to the Earth, and to our place on the Earth. They propel us forward into the future, carry us out of our past, and give us our stance in the present. Energetically, they function as accessories to the root chakra.

HEAD AND NECK: The head and neck contain the structures of the brain, and so generally are used for the higher mental functions that distinguish us from other animal species.

BACK: Our back receives the energies of our environment that we can't see coming toward us.

CHEST: The chest acts as a filter for the energies moving to and from our heart.

ABDOMEN: The abdomen filters the energies coming to and from our "gut"—our unconscious instincts and hunches.

HARA: The *Hara* is known in the Japanese culture as the center of power within the lower abdomen, a sphere of energy approximately 2-3 inches in diameter that sits 2-3 inches below the navel. The Chinese refer to this spot as the *tan tien*. It is the center of gravity and movement for all martial artists, and the center they draw from when performing forceful tasks (such as breaking boards, etc.). The Hara is said to be the center for our will to live in the physical body, the center that holds us in physical manifestation.

Within each of these body regions, there are common structures, such as

MUSCLES
BONES

LIGAMENTS AND TENDONS
BLOOD VESSELS
NERVES
JOINTS

There are also, depending on the region, more site specific structures such as:

EARS
EYES
NOSE
FINGERS
SHOULDER
KNEES
ETC.

If a body region tests positive, I then ask:

IS (the core answer) LOCATED IN A MORE SPECIFIC STRUCTURE OF THIS REGION?

If this tests positive, then I ask about each of the structures that are unique to the region, until I locate the most specific structure that tests "yes." Here again, the location and physiologic function of the structure may be indicative of the energy involved with our core answer. Or, as with the case of Nancy, the structure in that location may have been the site of some specific trauma in the past. For Nancy, both levels of the field involved with her headaches (emotional and mental) tested positive for the head and neck region, and then specifically the nose.

Of course, my quest for location can become extremely specific, such as asking about specific types of cells, molecules, atoms, etc.; but as a chiropractor, I don't often go down to those minute levels. Someone with a different type of healing specialty might be inclined to ask about other classifications of location, and there are many other possibilities. For example, if you are an acupuncturist, you may want to ask about specific meridians, or even specific acupuncture points.

In the case of my patient Sam, the chakras tested negative, so I went on and asked if the organs were related to his back pain. This tested positive, and the run-through of the organ locations had the liver test positive, making it clear that the cause of Sam's back pain was related to his liver. But related how, exactly? This is the starting place for my next series of questions. Once I know the location involved with my core answer, examining the other qualities of the energy held in that location may open up a completely new level of valuable information.

I can only find out by asking, so I muscle test this question:

DO WE NEED TO LOOK AT OTHER QUALITIES OF THE ENERGY IN (the location)?

If no, then I apparently have all the information I need, and can proceed to Step 3: **WORK WITH THE ENERGY** (Chapters 7-10). This was so with my patient Nancy, and in her case I concluded my muscle testing at this point, and proceeded to the business of working the energy that was located in her nose. The process of releasing and transforming the emotional and mental energies that she had been holding there is what revealed more about their nature. The fact that I was given no more advance information about the energy in Nancy's nose, other than its location, was an indication to me that she needed to experience the qualities of the energy firsthand.

A yes on this question indicates that the energy of our core answer has other specific qualities which, when examined, can inform us further about the nature of the answer. It also indicates that it would be helpful for us to have this information before we work the energy. The next series of questions are a framework for ascertaining these specific qualities.

DIRECTION

In Chinese medicine, energy is evaluated according to the polarities of yin and yang, hot and cold, deficient and excessive, and internal or external. For me, the most interesting of these is excess and deficiency. I begin my energy qualifying questions by examining this polarity, but I ask in terms of direction, i.e.: moving energy in or out of a location.

DO WE NEED TO MOVE ENERGY *IN* TO THIS LOCATION?
(Is the location deficient in energy?)

DO WE NEED TO MOVE ENERGY *OUT* OF THIS LOCATION?
(Does the location have an excess of energy?)

It's possible for both of these questions to test positive. If so, I like to follow up by asking which direction should be moved first.

BLOCK

Chinese medicine also focuses on the concept of blocked energy, based on the idea that it is the nature of energy to be in motion. When the movement of energy is blocked, stagnation results. Left unattended, stagnation eventually leads to dysfunction and disease. I check on the presence of a block in the location by asking:

IS THERE SOMETHING BLOCKING THE MOVEMENT OF ENERGY (*IN* or *OUT*) OF THIS LOCATION?

Energy Blocks are usually qualified as Entry or Exit Blocks, that is, a Block to energy moving *in* to the body or *out* of the body. If the energy needs to be moved *in* to the location, then any Block that may be present would naturally be an Entry Block. If energy needs to be moved *out* of the location, then any Block present would necessarily be an Exit Block.

With Sam *(CASE STUDY #2)*, I found that his liver needed energy moved *in*, and that there was an Entry Block present. The cause for Sam's back pain, in summary, was his liver, which was deficient in energy. His liver was deficient because its ability to intake energy was being blocked.

The search for further energetic qualifiers can now be applied to the energy that needs to be moved in or out, but can also be applied to the Block, that is, the energetic signature of the Block:

DO WE NEED TO KNOW MORE ABOUT THE QUALITIES OF THE ENERGY TO BE MOVED?

DO WE NEED TO KNOW MORE ABOUT THE QUALITIES OF THE BLOCK?

If the answer to both of these questions is "no", then there is no need to proceed further with qualifying questions. The location of the energy and the direction it needs to be moved (or the fact that it needs to be unblocked) may be all I need to know in order to go ahead and treat the patient. I can then skip ahead to Step 3: **WORK WITH THE ENERGY** (See Chapter 7-10).

If the answer to one or both questions is "yes", then I move further into the SEWLINE questions. Sam tested "yes" to both, which meant that there was more information available about the nature of the energy to be moved into his liver, as well as the nature of the Block in his liver.

The next group of questions is deceptively simple. Often, however, the answers provided are deliciously complex.

THE SIX W'S

IS THERE A *WHO* INVOLVED WITH THIS ENERGY?
IS THERE A *WHAT* INVOLVED?
IS THERE A *WHEN*?
IS THERE A *WHERE*?
IS THERE A *HOW*?
IS THERE A *WHY*?

With Sam, I had to apply these questions to the Block (the Block itself has an energetic signature, usually of a completely different quality than the energy it is blocking) as well as to the energy that was needed by the liver. The Block's energy tested as being related to the physical level of the field, and tested positive for the qualifier WHEN. The energy needing to be moved into the liver tested positive for the qualifiers WHO, and WHAT. You can see that the possible combinations of "yes" and "no" with these six qualifier questions involve rather advanced mathematics. Each "yes" answer requires further exploration, so let's examine them separately.

>
> **Patient/Other**
>
> **Individual/Group**
>
> **Known/Unknown**
>
> **Human/Non-Human**

(Diagram C – WHO)

If I get a "yes" to **WHO**, as a quality, I take it as an indication that the energy's signature can be compared to, or is related to, a person. Of course this makes me want to know who, exactly, the person is, which brings up the following questions:

IS THIS ENERGY RELATED TO THE PATIENT ONLY?

If yes, then for whatever reason, it needs to be emphasized that this energy is only related to the patient's own self.

If no, then the energy is obviously related to someone other than just the patient. We can find out who that is by asking:

IS THIS ENERGY RELATED TO A SINGLE INDIVIDUAL?

If no, then I must conclude that there are multiple individuals (a group) involved with this energy.

IS THE OTHER INDIVIDUAL/ GROUP INVOLVED CURRENTLY KNOWN TO THE PATIENT?

If yes, then I ask about specific categories of people, such as friends, family, co-workers, etc. If we are dealing with an individual, I go on to ask, and test, about specific people within that category until we nail it down to just one person.

If no, then I conclude that the energy is connected to someone unrelated and unknown to the patient. This can range from the mundane to the bizarre, and I find out who it is by asking:

IS THIS INDIVIDUAL/GROUP CURRENTLY ALIVE IN HUMAN FORM?

Yeah, I know, it's a pretty far-out question, but if I get a "yes", then it would seem that I should find out who this person or group is, in spite of their unfamiliarity to the patient. I often have to really think here, imagining who could fit into this category; my questions depend heavily on the patient's history and the personal issues contained therein.

If I get a "no" here, then I can inquire into categories of individuals or groups that might fit the description....not currently human. This includes, but is not limited to:

ANGELS
PAST LIFE RELATIONSHIPS OR SELVES

SIGNATURE ENERGY WORK

ALIENS
ATTACHED ENTITIES
ANIMALS
SPIRIT GUIDES
DECEASED INDIVIDUALS/GROUPS

All of these are categories that usually require special training to deal with, and it took me years of study to even begin to feel qualified. Even now I often refer patients to other practitioners who are more specialized and experienced than I in this.

```
┌─────────────────────┐
│                     │
│   Color             │
│                     │
│   Homeopathic       │
│   Remedy            │
│                     │
│   Flower Essence    │
│                     │
│   Other             │
│                     │
└─────────────────────┘
```

(Diagram D – WHAT)

A positive test for the **WHAT** quality indicates that the energy's signature is represented by, or related to, a thing—something of physical substance. I naturally want to explore the characteristics of this substance. There are many possibilities, but these are the categories of WHAT that I use most often:

IS THIS ENERGY RELATED TO A SPECIFIC COLOR?

If color tests positive, then I can check to see what is the specific color involved by telescoping through an almost infinitely long list of colors. The following are the most commonly used healing colors, and I usually find a match with one of these:

RED
ORANGE
YELLOW
GREEN
BLUE
INDIGO
VIOLET
GOLD
SILVER
WHITE

IS THIS ENERGY RELATED TO A HOMEOPATHIC REMEDY?

I am not a homeopathic physician, and have little training, other than my own limited personal experience, in homeopathic medicine. This is enough, however, to give me great respect for homeopathy. If this question tests positive, I funnel-test my collection of traditional homeopathic remedies, or funnel-test the lists of remedies that are found in the *Materia Medica*, a homeopathic reference book that lists all of the homeopathic remedies and their characteristics (see the Resources section at the end of the book). The characteristics of the remedy that test positive reflect the characteristics of the energy we are working with.

Here again is an example of how practitioners of different specialties may have another focus for their muscle-testing questions. Another class of subjects to be tested in the **WHAT** category might be herbal remedies, vitamins, minerals, or even different types of conventional medications. Each of these substances has its own unique set of characteristics, which may mirror the quality of energy of our core answer. One would need to be familiar with the characteristics of these substances to be able to make use of that information at this point in the SEWLINE testing.

IS THIS ENERGY RELATED TO A FLOWER ESSENCE?

Ah! One of my favorite subjects! Flower essences hold a vast array of possible characteristics, and offer such detailed and precise information that I find them almost unlimited in their usefulness to Signature Energy Work. There are many different types of flower essences: South American, Alaskan, English, etc. I am very drawn to the Flower Essence Society essences, which are North American flowers, but I encourage you to look into other types, and study the literature available on flower essences, starting with the work of Dr. Edward Bach, who originated the Bach Flower Remedies. I was first exposed to flower essences when I happened upon the work of Dr. Richard Gerber, M.D., who coined the term "vibrational medicine" in his book *Vibrational Medicine: New Choices for Healing Ourselves*. Dr. Gerber writes about the human being as a multidimensional energy system, with each person's energy forming a unique vibrational pattern that interacts with other energy systems. This interaction can enhance or inhibit the function of our bodies, and affect our overall health and well-being. Gerber saw consciousness as the main regulator of our vibrational pattern, and described the role of flower essences in this vibrational medicine model.

Gerber's writing led me to study the work of Dr. Bach, the "father" of flower essence therapy, as well as the work of Gurudas (*Flower Essences and Vibrational Healing*) and Machaelle Small Wright (*Flower Essences: Reordering Our Understanding and Approach to Illness and Health*) on the nature and uses of flower essences. What I found was that flower essences—homeopathic remedies made from flowers—embody energy patterns that accurately mirror emotional, mental and spiritual patterns of humans. Each flower remedy has its own unique energy pattern. In homeopathy this is called the "signature" of the remedy. Dr. Bach, and many others, catalogued detailed descriptions of the signatures of hundreds of different flowers. Flower essences are traditionally prescribed after a practitioner has thoroughly interviewed a patient to determine his predominant psychospiritual pattern, and matched this pattern with the signature of a particular flower. The corresponding flower remedy is then administered to treat the psychospiritual aspects of the patient's condition. I originally began experimenting with flower remedies by reversing this approach: I muscle-tested my patient to first determine which flower remedy was called for, and then studied the description of that flower's signature. Afterwards, I asked the patient questions about himself, to get a sense of his life and his feelings about his circumstances. What I found was that the signature of the flower *always* accurately described some important aspect of that patient's current pattern of thoughts, beliefs, and feelings -- that is to say, the signature of the flower accurately reflected the energetic signature of the patient's current problem or question. I realized that by finding what flower remedy the patient needed, I was shown the psychospiritual pattern he was working on.

If flower essences test positive at this point in the SEWLINE, it's because there is a flower remedy whose characteristics match the signature energy of our core answer. To find which flower is the match, I test through the collection of flower essences that I have in my office, funneling down to the specific flower that is involved. (See Appendix B: Funnel testing.) Let me digress slightly here, and at the same time give you a working example of the way that flower essences match the energetic signature of a core answer, by finishing my story about Margaret.

MARGARET (continued)

If you recall, we had framed the core question for Margaret's session as, "What is available for Margaret to learn in her relation with Jill?" (Jill being Margaret's co-worker who was going through terminal cancer, and who perhaps was reflecting for Margaret her relation with her own mother, who was in the end-stages of Alzheimer's disease.) Muscle-testing through the SEWLINE, I found that the answer to our question was related to all levels of the field, was located in the region of Margaret's lower back, and had qualities similar to the flower essence Gentian.

The region of the lower back is generally related to issues involving the concept of "support". This can range from problems with physical support, such as money, to feelings, ideas and beliefs about isolation, vulnerability, and the sense of supportedness/ supportiveness in one's life.

The signature characteristics of Gentian are described in the *Flower Essence Repertory,* written by Patricia Kaminski and Richard Katz (see Resources, for more information):

The soul can become strong and vibrant only by becoming resilient. Obstacles and problems test the soul's ability to respond, and to trust in the unfoldment of life. Those in need of Gentian become too easily discouraged and disheartened when problems and setbacks occur. Such souls view impediments as insurmountable problems, and are unable to discover solutions. The individual needs to learn that such vexing situations occur because they are exactly those lessons which are needed for growth and strength. Gentian gives encouragement, especially helping the soul to shift its mental perspective and see the long view. The doubting and skeptical qualities which the soul harbors are gradually transformed into deeper faith. Gentian flower essence helps the soul to acquire great inner fortitude and unwavering trust in the outcome of life events.[45]

    The lower back is about support, and Gentian is about faith, trust, seeing the long view, and giving encouragement. This is what the quantum level had to say about Margaret's question; as you can see, sometimes the tricky part is interpreting the information.

    I told Margaret that it seemed as though what was available for her to learn in relating to Jill was how to give support and encouragement. Jill was needing to develop her faith: her sense that everything is happening just as it should, and in the long run, from the "long view," everything is going to turn out OK. This is not an easy thing to convey to a person who is facing a terminal disease, but an extremely important thing to convey to a person who may be on the brink of stepping out of this life and into the next.

    Margaret said that she couldn't possibly see how she could give this to Jill: given Jill's self-isolating demeanor at work, and the limited nature of her relationship with Margaret, it just didn't seem like Jill would be very receptive to support and encouragement coming from Margaret.

    Yes, it was obviously going to be hard. But, I reminded her, the object of the exercise was for Margaret to *learn*. Learning is supposed to be challenging, and usually involves doing it awkwardly, and even badly, at the beginning. It's a process of gradual improvement and eventual mastery. (That's why there are so few masters: If it were easy, everyone would do it!) If Margaret wanted to master the fine art of giving support and encouragement to someone, she had a perfect opportunity to start the mastery process, in the form of Jill. Perhaps, I suggested, she could take what she learned with Jill, and apply it to her Mother.

```
Early Current Life

Past Life

Daily Current Life

Future Life
```

(Diagram E – WHEN)

A positive test for the **WHEN** quality indicates that the energetic signature or our answer is somehow related to a specific moment, or period, in time. The energetic dynamics in place during that time period reflect the dynamics of the energy of our answer. The specific details of when are found with the following questions:

IS THIS ENERGY RELATED TO A SPECIFIC TIME EARLIER IN THE PATIENT'S CURRENT LIFE?

If yes, then I can find the specific time period by testing in increasingly small groups of years, funneling down to the specific year. For example: age 0-10, age 10-20, etc.

IS THIS ENERGY RELATED TO A SPECIFIC PAST LIFE?

When this tests yes, it is an indication that it would be beneficial to explore the energetic dynamics of a previous lifetime, working on the premise that these dynamics are a mirror of the energy embodied in our core answer.

IS THIS ENERGY RELATED ONLY TO THE PATIENT'S CURRENT DAILY LIFE?

If yes, then I can break up the day into relevant pieces such as: mornings, while working, during meals, etc., and test each one until I find a positive indicator.

It's also possible that the energy is related to the patient's future self. This is rare, but it does happen.

IS THIS ENERGY RELATED TO THE PATIENT'S FUTURE LIFE?

If yes, I might ask about future periods within the current life, as well as actual future lives.

Let me summarize what I've said so far by taking you back to Sam.

SAM (continued)

If you recall, Sam's liver was deficient in energy due to a Block. The Block energy tested as being physical in nature, and had been in place since he was 7 years old (WHEN). The energy that was being blocked, that needed to move *in* to his liver, was emotional, characterized by the flower essence Mariposa Lily (WHAT), and was related to his mother (WHO). I explained these findings to Sam, then read aloud to him the description of Mariposa Lily, as found in the *Flower Essence Repertory*:

The ability of the human soul to show nurturing and caring attention for others depends very much on whether it has received such nurturing itself. Each person should be able, as a divine birthright, to receive maternal love and unconditional support as a young infant and child. Many souls are deprived of a positive relationship to the mother. Especially in the modern world, cultural conditions de-humanize the relationship of the infant to the mother through birthing and child-rearing practices. Further deprivation may result from family trauma, divorce, economic hardship, or extreme situations of abuse, abandonment, and neglect. If the soul is crippled in its early relationship to the feminine, it feels cold and empty inside, and at its core, experiences itself as unloved and unwanted. The maturation process into adulthood is usually distorted – for males a rejection of or hostility to the feminine, and for females an alienation from their own mothering instincts. Mariposa Lily helps such souls heal this trauma by coming to terms with the painful past. It is an extremely important remedy, not only for infants and children, but also for many phases of adult therapy and positive parenting. Despite the wounding which may have occurred through an imperfect human mother, the soul can learn to forgive and heal, by experiencing the presence of the divine or archetypal mother who embraces the entire human family with gentle mercy and nurturing. This ability of the soul to feel and embrace the warm, loving presence of the maternal is the very important gift of the Mariposa Lily.

I asked Sam to describe his mother to me, reminding him that the Mariposa Lily pattern was hers, and not necessarily his. He explained that his mother had been born in a very small town, the fourth child of five children, and the only girl. Her own mother had died before she could remember, at which time her father had then taken her back to the large city where he was born, many miles away. He left her, for months at a time, to live with a succession of unfamiliar and indifferent families. Because her father was something of a gambler and often did not have money to pay for her upkeep, she rarely stayed too long in any one place. This was her childhood. She had barely become a young woman, living on her own in a small boarding house, when the country broke out into civil war. There was shooting and shelling in the streets of the city; she lost friends, co-workers, and neighbors. No one was safe. She was desperate to escape the nightly bombings and horrific violence, and finally left the city, alone, returning to the town of her birth. She found refuge on the farm of her eldest brother, but again couldn't stay there long, this time because her brother's wife became very jealous. Sam smiled and said that his mother was considered quite a beauty when she was young, and apparently her sister-in-law didn't appreciate feeling like the ugly duckling in her own home. Being a young woman living alone in a small town, she was desperate for some type of security. Sam's father came from a very powerful family in the town, and seemed to offer the type of stability she craved. So she married the doctor, and soon found out that the doctor was not a very astute businessman, nor a very devoted husband. She spent the next 30 years scrimping for money, living in their small house, in their small town, a very lonely and unhappy woman.

This description correlated perfectly with the Mariposa Lily. His mother had been deeply wounded by losing her mother. She felt unwanted and unloved from her earliest memory, and this painfully wounded child was what she projected outward into the world whenever she felt unhappy. And she usually projected it toward the people to whom she felt closest.

"You don't love me" is a very negative energy to be faced with every day. Sam's father quickly became immune to it, and stopped spending much time at home. Sam had nowhere else he could go. He had the limited understanding and resources of a child, so he did what "good" children do. He swallowed his mother's beliefs and feelings—lock, stock, and barrel. And then he made it all about him; all his fault, all his resposibility. In his mind, he was the one who didn't love her enough, he was the one causing her pain, and he was the one who should fix it.

Our muscle-testing had indicated that Sam began blocking the negative emotional energy coming from his mother at 7 years of age, so I asked him what particular event he could recall from that time in his life. He shrugged, as if trying to flick the question away with his shoulders, and then reluctantly explained.

Because he lived in a very small town, there was no school nearby. His mother taught him his alphabet and numbers, reading and basic math, at home. He was a pretty fast learner, and by the time he was 7, his mother had taught him everything that her own very limited education could provide for him. By this time he was also the apple of his mother's eye. Because his father was almost always out of the house, occupied with his practice or his small-town cronies, his mother often looked to Sam for attention and affection. From a very young age, as young as he could remember, he was her protector. He always took care of her when she was lonely, afraid, or ill, which was often. He recalled many times running to his father's office, terrified because his mother was having one of her "faint spells." She would tell Sam that she thought she was about to die, and to go fetch the doctor. Usually his father would just scowl and tell Sam that he was too busy, and that his mother was just being hysterical. Sometimes he would send Sam back with a nurse, who would sit with his mother until she felt better.

When he was 7, Sam had to leave his mother to go off to school in the next town, riding the bus daily on his own. In the small world of his home, he was the perfect son. In the larger world he was, of course, a complete mama's boy. Placed in a class of children that were older than he was, because of his mother's diligence at home, he was the smallest boy in his classroom. His classmates teased him mercilessly, and the teasing escalated into beatings. He was too small to defend himself, and the teachers didn't seem to see what was going on. Sam still felt, some 50 years later, a tremendous sense of shame and anger about this. He still saw himself as weak. This certainly explained why the liver was the site of the blocking energy. The liver is the processor of anger and shame, so naturally it would be affected.

I asked Sam why his mother hadn't intervened in this situation. Did she not speak to the teachers, or to the principal of the school? (I pictured myself jumping down the principal's throat with fingernails bared if he didn't get those thugs off *my* baby.) He said that he never told her about it. He didn't know why.

Wow.

Of course he didn't tell her. He was her protector; it never occurred to him that she should be protecting *him*. The collision of her needs and his had paralyzed him, and his ability to seek protection. The anger at his abusers, and the shame at being abused, became bottled up in his liver. From that time forward, he used that angry liver heat to block her emotional projections - her feelings of being unloved and unwanted (the negative qualities of Mariposa Lily). This was the only way he could find to protect himself. Now, whenever he was very stressed by the circumstances of his adult life—when he needed a little nurturing and caring (the positive Mariposa Lily qualities)—the liver would ignite again, blocking his ability to take in these energies and triggering his back pain and mouth ulcers.

Self-Discovery, Self-Healing

This would be a good time for me to mention another important category of patient that I treat. That would be me. I contend that every patient who enters my office has something to teach me, something to offer in terms of my own personal Signature Energy Work. Sam was definitely one of those. His description of his mother, and the dynamic between them in which he was expected, at a very young age, to give her the parental-type nurturing that she never had, resonated strongly with me. His response to that dynamic, and the consequences of that response in his body, were so similar to my own that it was impossible not to notice. In effect, he cut himself off from the emotional energy of his mother, thus leaving him to continue on his own, unmothered—at least at the emotional level. This should have been my signal to do a little work on my own "mother issues". Should have.

Coincidentally, I woke up a few days later with a cold.

I really hate having colds, or any kind of illness for that matter. It's so inelegant, and it really shatters the whole "I'm your doctor, I know everything about being healthy" myth. My ego adores that myth. Anyway, I definitely woke up with a full-blown cold. And to add coincidental insult to injury, it also happened to be my mother's birthday. It was obviously time for me to check in with my own signature energy, to find out what was going on. I muscle tested myself (See Appendix D: Surrogate and Self-Testing), and found that the energy related to my cold was at the mental level, and the location of the energy involved was in my heart (ORGAN), which needed some help releasing (moving *out*) this mental energy. The energy to be released was related to the (WHAT) flower essence Goldenrod, and needed to be released through the sixth chakra (WHERE). I also needed to look at the WHY of this energy, which I do in Chapter 10.

This little cold of mine illustrates the importance of good "energy hygiene;" also known as self-care. If you are going to practice Signature Energy Work, or any work, for that matter, that involves moving into other people's energetic field, you are going to experience the phenomena of resonance. My own issues, those in resonance with the issues of the person I am working with, will be triggered. That's a good thing, because it is what allows my intuition to work, and because it brings to my attention the things in my own self that are in need of healing. It can also be a bad thing if I don't pursue my own healing work: examining, discovering, and cleaning up my issues when they are triggered (and me "catching" a cold is a perfect example of the consequences of that). The resonance phenomena can also be a problem if I hold a patient's unhealed energy in my own field, as a mechanism to heal them, without later coming back and cleaning that out of my field. We must, **MUST**, have a regular cleansing and self-healing routine in place in order to do this work effectively without eventually making ourselves sick with other people's energy stored in our own system. Self-care is obviously an art that I myself am still trying to master.

If **WHERE** tests positive, as in my own example above, it tells me that the energy of our core answer is related to a place—the energy is *coming from* somewhere, or is *going to* somewhere. These are my next questions:

SHOULD THE ENERGY GO FROM THIS LOCATION TO ANOTHER PLACE?

SHOULD THE ENERGY COME FROM ANOTHER PLACE TO THIS LOCATION?

One of these two questions will test yes. I can find out where the energy is going to/coming from by employing the original **LOCATION** questions. In my own example above, the WHERE energy was going to another place, specifically the 6th chakra.

When the **HOW** quality tests positive, it's an indication that the energy needs to be qualified by the patient himself, before the energy is moved. The patient needs to perceive, in whatever way he can, how the energy presents itself. This requires the patient to use a little imagination, go inside, and "see" the energy. This might mean actually seeing, on an inner level, how the energy looks, but also includes perceiving how the energy feels, moves, smells, sounds. I ask the patient to use all five senses if possible, and notice any colors, words, sounds, temperature, shape, size, texture, symbols or feelings that go with the energy. You'd be surprised at how perceptive people can be, given a little encouragement.

If the quality of **WHY** tests positive, then we need to understand the purpose behind the energy; why it is there. I like to have the patient "go inside" and converse with the energy, asking the energy what its purpose is, in relation to the patient, and listening to the response that comes up.

If we are qualifying a blocking energy, and the WHY qualifier shows up, this indicates that the Block has a purpose that needs to be examined. The purpose was probably relevant at the time the Block was put in place, but perhaps has now become obsolete. We often place energetic Blocks in our field as a defense mechanism, in response to something that feels threatening to us in our environment. Frequently these protective Blocks are created unconsciously, or from the limited point of view of the child. If such a Block is removed without examining its purpose, the patient will be left feeling unprotected, and most probably will just recreate the Block. When examined consciously, from the adult point of view, the Block is often found to be obsolete, its original purpose having long since become irrelevant. The energy used to sustain the Block can then be safely released, and the Block removed, or the energy can be transformed, and given a new purpose that is more relevant to current circumstances - such as acting as a filter rather than a Block.

If we are qualifying an energy that is to be moved *in* to the patient, and the WHY qualifier tests positive, it indicates the need for the patient to understand the purpose of the energy to be moved in, before the energy can enter. This is often so that the patient can commit himself to *using* the energy, once he has brought it into place.

When we are qualifying an energy that is to be moved *out* of the patient, we need to understand its purpose before moving it out, perhaps because the patient is still attached to holding the energy, and doesn't understand why it needs to be released, or perhaps because the energy's purpose is not something that we want to let loose in the environment without a little alteration beforehand.

* * * * * * * * *

SIGNATURE ENERGY WORK

Once all of the qualities of the energy in our location have been revealed, I am ready to move to the next step in Signature Energy Work, which is working with the energy. I make sure to write down all the information that I have picked up in my SEWLINE testing (see Appendix G: SEWLINE Report of Findings), so that I can use it to form a clear, multi-dimensional picture of the signature energy pattern of our core answer. This picture guides me toward an accurate understanding of the relation between the core question and the core answer, which then guides us in designing an appropriate energy-work treatment.

CHAPTER 7

STEP THREE: WORK WITH THE ENERGY

SAM (continued)

As I gently but firmly began to move my hands into his liver area, I explained to Sam that it was time for him to stop blocking the emotional energy of mother. He laughed shallowly and explained that his mother had died several years ago. Yes, I concurred, unblocking himself to *his* mother's emotional energy would do him little good, by the way, even if she were still living. What he needed now was to open up to the emotional nurturing of the archetypal mother, the warm and unconditionally loving energy that is the ideal of Mother.

I explained that eventually it becomes necessary for each of us to look to a higher source of emotional mothering than just our own human mother's. As children, our mother provides us with the general sense that everything is OK, that we are taken care of, that there is a wiser, more powerful intelligence in charge of our welfare, and that this powerful intelligence is guiding us toward our highest potential. Somewhere along the way to adulthood we have to shift this natural human expectation of "mothering" from our actual human mother, to our spiritual Mother—the benevolent intelligence of the universe, God, Goddess, Spirit, our own Higher Self, Destiny, etc. (depending on one's spiritual orientation).

Without the general sense that we are protected and guided, we may be left with a deep and constant undercurrent of fear. Sam had been disconnected from this sense of being "mothered" since he was 7 years old, effectively blocking his ability to shift to a higher sense of "Mother". I told Sam, bluntly, that now was the time for him to start shifting. He looked at me hard, as though fully measuring my intention, and then said, emphatically, that he had absolutely no idea how to do that.

Of course not, I reassured him. The natural model for this type of shift should be his own parents, who, while Sam was a child, would be gradually developing their own mature sense of Mother as their lives progressed, and their own spiritual experiences and understandings took shape. This would have allowed Sam to witness their shifting process, thus giving him a natural familiarity with it. But Sam's father had rarely been available to him as a model for anything, and his mother had never made the shift herself, which is of course why Sam had been coerced into being her protector.

Faith, a sense of trust in and connection with a larger source of guidance and purpose, is often like an undeveloped muscle that just needs to be exercised. Sam's assignment, then, was to *practice the feeling* of faith. In order to accomplish that, he would first need to spend some time *thinking* about the nature of faith, for him personally: what it would be like to know that everything was going along perfectly, as planned by a higher level of intelligence. With that definition in mind, he then had to learn to stop himself when he felt stressed, or when his liver or back was hurting—because those were sure signs of stress—and practice *feeling* as if he was part of an elegant but yet-to-be-revealed plan. He could then put his energy into understanding the nature and validity of this plan, instead of resisting it, or worse, sabotaging it with negativity and doubt.

Sam confessed his tendency to get very angry when things start to go wrong for him. His anger might be triggered by a small event, but it would then escalate into thoughts about how everything *always* goes badly for him, and extrapolating from his current situation into the fear that everything would soon fall apart and leave him in whatever worst possible scenario came to mind. I pointed out that he obviously was going to need a lot of practice, and that it would probably help for him to look at the people around him, and see how they manage to stay calm and positive in difficult situations. He could follow their example, and the more he practiced, the stronger the "faith" muscle would become.

The Work of Transformation

The "work" of Signature Energy Work is about moving and transforming energy. We can analyze the energy of our core answer with the SEWLINE questions, bringing to our conscious attention as many of the qualities of the answer's energetic signature as possible. Sometimes this is as far as we need to go: understanding the answer. But we have the opportunity to go farther.

The relationship between the core question and its answer represents a habitual pattern (of thoughts, feelings, actions, and/or beliefs) that is limiting us in some way, and is presenting itself for change. We can literally change the form of this pattern, by replacing it with a new pattern, based on the energy of the core answer. If, according to our understanding of quantum physics, everything is energy, and takes on physical form only according to our observation of the energy—how we see it, how we feel about it, the meaning we attach to it—then we can actually change the physically manifesting form of an energy by changing how we observe it. In Sam's case, we wanted to change the energy that was manifesting in the form of back spasms and mouth ulcers, into something more comfortable. Maybe even something useful.

Direct Access: The Internal Path

There are a myriad of energy-work modalities and techniques out there, and almost as many teachers, many better than I, to show you how to use them. It is not my aim to sell you on any particular energy-work technique, but I will be mentioning some of the techniques that I like to use, if only as a means to illustrate a point.

All energy-work techniques fall into two basic categories: direct techniques, and indirect techniques. According to Gay Hendricks, Ph.D., in his book *At the Speed of Life: A New Approach to Personal Change Through Body-Centered Therapy*, a direct technique is one in which the patient places his non-judgmental, conscious awareness on the problem.

Of course this is much easier said than done.

In order to arrive at a "non-judgmental, conscious awareness" of the problem, we must take what Gregg Braden calls the path of "internal technology,"[46] or the *internal path*. The basis for the internal path is, once again, the understanding derived from quantum physics that form follows thought: we create our reality with our consciousness. The core question (or the core problem related to the question) is examined from the inside, implying that the problem is not happening *to* us—imposed on us by some outside, external force—but rather *through* us. We are creating, or expressing, the problem based on who we are: our feelings, thoughts, actions, and beliefs—our consciousness. As such, we are not just seeking a solution for the problem, but rather we are seeking to understand the meaning of the problem, as a means to understand who we are—our own purpose and meaning; the meaning behind our thoughts, feelings, beliefs, and actions. We seek to understand the problem, ultimately, as a means to understand ourselves: to elevate our level of consciousness, and therefore elevate the quality of our reality. The problem resolves as soon as we understand its message for us, because its single purpose is to deliver that message to us.

Direct/internal techniques focus on *creating growth* of the body-mind. At the highest level of Signature Energy Work, this growth is created in the patient as well as the practitioner. The nonjudgmental awareness of *both* the patient and the practitioner can be placed on the problem. As we glean information from the SEWLINE, the true nature of the core answer becomes clearer, allowing us to become fully aware of its energy: how the problem it represents was constructed, and how it affects us. I say "us," because my patient's core questions and answers offer me, the practitioner, an opportunity to focus my own conscious awareness on the same energy pattern in *my* signature energy field; on the same thread as it is woven into my own energetic garment. I refer to this as direct/internal energy work because the patient uses the core question as an opportunity to "go inside": to focus his nonjudgmental, conscious awareness on his Self-limiting energy patterns. In addition, I can, if I choose to, acknowledge the resonance between my patient's Self-limiting patterns and my own—between his signature energy and mine—and capitalize on that resonance. It is the resonance of our energies that allows both the patient and the practitioner to focus their intention for change directly on the problem pattern. And the pattern changes in both of us.

Indirect Application: The External Path

An indirect energy work technique is one that moves energy *for* the patient: I apply the technique to the patient (or the patient applies the technique to himself), and the patient receives the energy-work *from* the practitioner (or from the technique) without any active, conscious participation in the process. The practitioner performs the healing techniques *on* the patient, without attempting to focus his, and/or the patient's, conscious awareness on *understanding*: understanding the problem—its meaning, its purpose for the patient—or the relationship between the problem and the patient—how he has created the problem in order to effect change. Indirect techniques are based on the path of "external technology," wherein we see our problem as coming from some external source, which is intruding into our body and creating an illness or a dysfunction. We seek to change that external source so that it no longer causes our problem. I employ my own repertoire of indirect/external energy work techniques—chiropractic adjustment, neuromuscular massage, myofascial unwinding, etc.—on my patients. I use, and encourage my patients to use, other indirect energy work techniques, such as yoga, Tai Chi, qi gong, or pranic breathing (and there are many, many more), as part of a regular self-healing practice. These are techniques that move energy; they may move energy in a general way, or they may move a specific energy related to a specific problem, but do not require, nor necessarily create, any conscious awareness of the problem. Indirect/external techniques focus on *restoring balance* to the body.

An Integrated Path

Signature Energy Work allows for the patient and the practitioner to combine both direct/internal and indirect/external techniques, using them simultaneously, and mutually. The energy-balancing power of any indirect/external energy work technique—whether it be a modality employed by a practitioner, such as chiropractic, acupuncture, surgery, soul retrieval, chakra balancing, etc., or a self-directed technique such as Reiki, yoga, nutrition, or just a good walk in the park—is enormously amplified by the addition of a direct/internal technique.

And the opposite also applies: the direct transformation of an energetic pattern, and the integration of a new pattern in to the signature energy field, is amplified by the addition of an indirect/external energy work technique to the process. The core question, and its answer, catalyzes a conscious, direct, and active exploration of the nature of the Self-limiting energy pattern, which allows us to choose, and intend, a new pattern. Anyone can connect this intention to an indirect/external energy work session, and amplify the power of such a session.

Even more potent is the power of patient and practitioner working together, connecting their active, combined attention to the core question, and their clear, mutually-held intention for pattern-transformation—for the manifestation of a new pattern of being—during the energy work process. The resonant power of two people combined is greater than the power of each working alone. The addition of the practitioner's resonance—with the problem pattern, as well as with the chosen replacement pattern—amplifies the power of transformation focused on the pattern, and assists in integrating the new pattern into the signature energy fields of *both* patient *and* practitioner. This transformation and integration of energy is again amplified by the addition of an indirect/external technique to the energy work session.

The indirect energy-work techniques that I am most inclined toward usually include some type of body-work. I am trained in a hands-on profession, so touch is not only a familiar modality for me, it is an important one. There are many effective non-touching indirect modalities as well, and these can successfully be used alone, or in combination with body-work. Indirect techniques, both hands-on and hands-off, can be interwoven beautifully with direct techniques in the course of a single energy work session. By way of example, let me finish the stories of my patients Sam and Maria.

SAM (the final piece)

I once again asked Sam to lie face down so that I could access the area of his spine that is related neurologically to his liver, and work on the physical energy of the block held in his mid-back muscles. I put a few drops of the Mariposa Lily essence on my hands, and began to probe the muscular trigger points - the knots of tension and blocked, stagnant energy - in his back. As I worked, I asked him to focus on letting go of the blocking energy held in this area; the anger and shame, as well as the belief that he was unprotected, and so must constantly defend himself. I instructed him to let this blocking energy flow outward, off of his body and into my hands, where I could collect it for him, and dispose of it properly. He breathed deeply, allowing my hands to move deeper into the tissues, releasing the tension held there. Once the release felt complete, I told him that it was time to set an intention for the type of "mothering" energy he would now like to experience and contain in this area. After giving him some time to clarify this intention in his mind, I then asked him once again to engage his breath with his intention: using his breath as an energetic pump, he inhaled his new "Mother" energy toward himself, and then exhaled it into his back and his liver, filling the area with feelings of safety, nurturing, and love.

I have seen Sam since that visit for other problems, but his severe mid-back spasms and mouth ulcers have never recurred to any significant extent. He told me that when he feels his back start to tighten up, or the familiar hot pain in his mouth begins to threaten, he tries to relax and look for the value in his current circumstances – explore what they might be teaching him, rather than assume that something is "wrong". This always allows his symptoms to fade.

MARIA (continued)

As you may recall, Maria, the dancer, was questioning her lack of success in her work. She had also mentioned symptoms that sounded like tachycardia (rapid heart beat). My muscle testing showed that her "unsuccessful in work" pattern was coming from the spiritual level of her being, and was located in the heart chakra. Further testing showed that the heart chakra energy involved had WHO qualities, as well as WHAT qualities, related to it. The WHO aspect tested as someone that Maria did not know, and that was coming to her from another lifetime. The WHAT aspect tested as being represented by a flower essence, Wild Rose. This energetic pattern was to be moved *out* of Maria's heart chakra.

Maria was a new patient for me. I had never seen her before, so I was reluctant to plunge so quickly into the far fringes of reality that dealing with a spiritual pattern—coming from someone in another plane of existence—would likely take us. These are not widely accepted clinical concepts, so I usually prefer to establish more rapport with a person before marching into such expansive levels. Luckily, expansion was something that Maria was familiar with. As soon as I began to explain my findings to her, she closed her eyes and took what appeared to be a huge sigh of relief. With tears in her eyes, she explained that she had often had the feeling that the situation was somehow beyond her; as if it were coming from somewhere other than just her self.

Somewhere and someone.

I looked up the *Flower Essence Repertory* description of Wild Rose. It reads as follows:

> The Wild Rose essence first developed by Dr. Bach addresses broad and important soul themes of motivation and interest in the world and in others. In this way, it is similar to the California Wild Rose. However, this English Rose specifically

addresses the type of resignation in the soul which depletes one's vitality. Physical incarnation in a body is an experience fraught with difficulty and struggle, and for the Wild Rose personality the effort hardly seems worth making. Such apathy suppresses the soul's interest in life, and cuts off the individual from his or her inner sources of healing. This essence is very helpful for those who linger in long, drawn-out illness, and who seem to recover only fitfully and slowly. Wild Rose restores the vital forces of the soul, particularly its connection to the physical body and to the physical world, helping the individual regain an interest in earthly life. This essence teaches that life is a sacred and precious opportunity which the soul must make every effort to embrace, if it is to find the true meaning of love and physical incarnation.

In this case, I decided not to read, nor even explain to Maria the characteristics of the flower essence. I knew that some visionary "regression" type work was called for, since we were working in the spiritual level, and in such cases I prefer to give the patient as few details as possible in advance, in order not to "lead" them into any particular experience. I guided Maria into a deeper state of relaxation, and then instructed her to go to the time and place where this problematic energy pattern originated. Maria is a very creative and artistic person, so traveling across the fluid boundaries of individual personality was very easy for her.

She immediately found herself in the body of a woman who she described as having dark eyes and dark hair. The woman was dressed in a long colorful dress, with brightly colored ribbons attached to it. Maria said it felt very much as if she were a gypsy: very beautiful and sensual, full of vitality, and passionately self-expressive. I smiled to myself at what an apt description of a "Wild Rose" that was. A moment later, the scene changed, and she was in the same body, but years later

She's old now. Her clothes are the same, but faded. She's kind of ragged and disheveled, and she seems very confused. I hear her saying over and over, "He did this to me; it's his fault." It's like she's lost all of her beauty, all her color and passion for life because of "him." She seems to be ill, and very disconnected. She seems...lost.

I asked Maria if there was anything else we needed to know about this scene. After a few moments hesitation, she shook her head. I then instructed her to move forward in time, to the last moment of this woman's life, just before she died. Again she went silent, as if searching, and finally said, softly,

I don't think she died. She just stayed like that, wandering around confused, and kind of stuck.

Oh boy. This is the kind of answer that makes no objective sense, definitely the type of moment when you cling tightly to your belief in the power of your intuition. I mulled over my next question silently, trying to understand what, exactly, I was dealing with here: an incomplete past life? An energy attachment from another life? An unwillingness, on Maria's part, to take responsibility for her current problems, being projected into some sort of "alternate personality?" I'm still not convinced that these distinctions really matter, but my intuition said that I needed to take the situation very seriously, and that I needed to help this energy move out. I spoke firmly to Maria, telling her that it was apparent that this gypsy woman needed to move on, and I asked her if she was ready to let the old woman go.

Maria started to breathe faster, as if she didn't understand my question. She replied vaguely that her heart was beating rapidly, and her back was hurting. She sounded distant, and I could hear an edge of fear in her voice. I knew that more questions were impossible, for now, and that it was time to step in and move this Wild Rose energy. My intuition told me to recruit some help here, not just for my own sense of safety, but also for Maria's. She seemed to be slipping into the emotional state of this old woman, and needed something that would give her some assurance and clarity in order to proceed. I decided that, given Maria's religious and cultural background, it would be appropriate to call in some angelic helpers.

    I spoke in my most authoritative "doctor" tone, saying that I was now calling into the room with us the presence of Archangel Michael. Maria smiled, and her confusion shifted instantly. I told her I was asking Michael to bring with him his entourage of Helper Angels. I requested that they surround this old gypsy woman, and her energy, with an impenetrable net of light that would separate the gypsy's energy from Maria's, and contain the gypsy's energy within it. Immediately Maria's energy seemed to elevate; she was smiling blissfully now, and her posture had shifted from fearful to confident. She was obviously familiar with Archangel Michael, and his power (Archangel Michael is traditionally depicted, in Judeo-Christian lore, as carrying a large, flaming sword, and is considered to be the Archangel in charge of fighting the forces of darkness). I explained to Maria that we would take care of the gypsy woman in a moment, but first I wanted Maria to see why this woman was connected with her. What was it in Maria's signature energy that resonated with this gypsy's, and so attracted the gypsy to her?
I asked Maria to take a look at her own energy, at the circumstances of her current life, to see what was similar to the gypsy's. She relaxed and took a few deep breaths, then quickly opened her eyes and looked at me,

Well, I haven't told you this, but there's this man...

It turns out that Maria had been feeling pretty stuck lately. She was living in a small apartment building in a not-very-good part of town, and had become physically intimate with the owner of the building. He said that he sympathized with her financial problems, and so made her the "resident manager" of the building. As such, she was responsible for addressing any problems that arose with the other tenants in the building, and in return he held her rent at a stable level, with no yearly increases. She explained that there was currently an active drug dealer living in the building, as well as a middle-aged man who lived, and perpetually fought, with his elderly mother—frequently threatening physical violence. And then there was her upstairs neighbor who played in a rock band, and spent many nights practicing, loudly, into the small hours of the morning. The owner would not allow her to call the authorities to deal with these people, and refused to evict them. He would tell her that she should handle them, berating her for not being smart enough, or brave enough to do so effectively. He told her she was weak, a failure, and becoming too old and ugly for anyone to want her. He disappeared for weeks at a time, showing up suddenly with small gifts of money: $20 here and there, just enough to take her through this week's financial crisis, but never enough to really do her any good. She was afraid to stop seeing him, even though she felt constantly degraded by him, because she felt that she couldn't afford to pay more rent elsewhere, and she didn't want to lose his occasional gifts.

As with the old gypsy, this man was slowly wearing away her vitality and her sense of self. She too was deeply in need of moving on, but felt confused and afraid. She had become increasingly resigned to living in this powerless state, lacking the strength to struggle against it. As a result of this, she was becoming more and more disconnected from her passion in life, her dance.

I told Maria that I was now going to ask Michael and some of his helpers to escort the old gypsy to a place in the light, a place where she could be cared for and healed, and from which she could progress with her own evolution. I explained that I was going to make some adjustments that would disconnect the gypsy's energy from Maria. I put some Wild Rose essence on my hands, and began to work the trigger points around Maria's heart, both on the chest and on the middle back. I made some adjustments to her neck and back, and then moved up to the trigger points around the head and neck. Again I invoked the assistance of the Helper Angels, to cleanse the areas in Maria's signature energy that had been holding the gypsy's energy, and to move healing energy into them. I sat, holding Maria's head in my hands, until it felt like this process was complete.

    We can conjecture all over the place about the nature of this gypsy woman, but in the end, it only really matters who she was for Maria. She said it felt like the gypsy was her own self, or an aspect of herself, but in something like a parallel universe. It was as though she had come to a crossroad in some distant time, and the gypsy was who she would have been if she had taken the other road. She realized now that she was getting dangerously close to that same, dark road, by depending on a man who obviously didn't have her best interest at heart, and by believing she had no other choice. She admitted that she was afraid to move out of her apartment, but could see it was imperative she do so. She just wasn't sure *how* to do it.

    I told her she didn't need to know how; she just needed to know what.

    Maria just blinked at me, unsure of what I meant. People usually just blink when I say that.

    I explained to Maria my theory of manifestation. I call it a theory, in spite of the fact that it's based on very ancient principles, because I think it's important for everyone to prove these principles to themselves; for themselves. I gave her my version (yes, my simplified version) of how manifestation works.

Manifestation: Quantum Reality into Physical Reality

One of the general purposes of physical life is physical creation, that is, to draw energy from its quantum, purely potential state, and manifest it into physical form. (We each have some specific thing, or things, that we came into life to manifest, but that's another subject for further discussion.) The Universe will supply us with whatever we need to create the physical reality we want; all we have to do is ask. Our job is to know what we want to manifest, the Universe is in charge of how it manifests.

Aspiration

The first step to manifestation, then, is to know what you really want. This involves **thinking,** that is, engaging the mental body and pulling mental energy into the process in a clear and sustained manner. Believe it or not, this is often the hardest part. I am amazed at how often I ask people what they want, and they have absolutely no idea. I attribute this to the way in which most of us were raised, which essentially consisted of being taught not to want anything. Disappointment, as a child, at not getting what you want, or worse, having unbearable strings attached to what you get, eventually make it not worth asking for anything. While your parents had dozens of their own issues attached to giving you what you asked for, the Universe is much less personal. There are three basic stipulations here, and these are mine, based on my own experience, rather than on any cosmic prohibitions:

1. You don't want to manifest something that takes away someone else's right or ability to pursue what they want. I say, "don't want to" because if

you ask for these things and get them, you will eventually regret it. The corollary to this is: you don't need to. You can have what you want without taking anything away from anyone.

2. You also don't want to manifest things that are in direct conflict with each other. For example, you can't be in two places at the same time, so if you find yourself asking for a promotion at work, and at the same time asking for a nice, long vacation, this may get you a net result of nothing.

3. Be concise: Ask for your highest possible aspiration, expressed in the fewest possible words. This is a very important concept, so let's use Maria's situation to illustrate.

It seemed to me that Maria wanted, among other things, a new home to live in. This is a fairly specific request, but perhaps not very concise. In order to manifest your highest possible aspiration, you need to know not only what you want, but why you want it.

Inspiration

The question of "why you want it" leads us to the second step in manifestation, which involves **feeling**: drawing input from the emotional body. What are the fundamental feelings that you want to feel in your life, that having what you ask for can help you to generate? Or, better said, what is the feeling that you want to get from having what you want?

Maria wanted a new home in order to feel safe (away from drug-dealing neighbors), and to feel independent (from her landlord/lover). I pointed out that it appeared she was also seeking to feel empowered (in touch with her own personal power, and the power of her personal gifts), accomplished (using her gifts fully in order to make a meaningful contribution), and connected (to her Source, as well as to her true self). These are essential elements of happiness, the antithesis of depression. Maria nodded her head emphatically in agreement: this was definitely what she wanted—empowerment, accomplishment, connectedness.

In order to feel empowered, we need to know what our personal gifts are. I told Maria that she was lucky, in that she already knew what her gift was: to dance beautifully, gracefully, and passionately. For many of my patients, the work of discovering their gifts, or just discovering the idea that they might actually have a gift, has to be done first.

In order to feel accomplished, we need to know what is the contribution that we wish to make with our gifts. Maria didn't have to think about that one very long either. She wanted to contribute a sense of beauty and sensuality to the people who witnessed her dance; she wanted to lead them to their own inner sense of beauty and sensuality.

Finally, in order to feel a sense of connection with our deeper self, as well as our Source, we have to personally experience that connection. And how to do that?

A profound question, and, as they say, there are many roads up the mountain. One way is to take an honest and thorough inventory of yourself and see what it is that you really want, what it is that inspires you to life. Ask your Source to provide it for you, and when it comes to you, take it. Let it be for you: use it, and make your contribution with it. Let it teach you, let it challenge you, let it show you who you are. Use that information to ask for your next thing.

So simple.

Maria wanted a new home where she could feel safe and independent, in order to dance beautifully, gracefully, and passionately, as a means to inspire a sense of beauty and sensuality in the people around her, as well as to connect to the beauty and sensuality of her own Self.

Now that's concise.

Reception

And this brings me to the third step in manifestation: **doing**. Taking action. Manifestation takes practice, and like anything, the more you practice, the better you get at it. When we practice manifestation, we practice thinking about what we want, and just as important, we practice feeling what we want. In Maria's case, she practices seeing herself in her new home, feeling safe and independent. She practices feeling the sense of power and accomplishment that comes when she dances in front of an audience that understands her intention, and swells with passion and beauty in response to her movements. She practices feeling absolutely connected to the passionate core of her being that generates that beauty; her own Source.

In order to receive what we've requested, we need to practice, but we must also insure that we're in the right place, and the right frame of mind, to be able to recognize our creation when it shows up. In essence, we have to *become* what we *ask* for: we have to act as if we already have it by attuning our thoughts, our habits, and our expectations to the assumption that what we are asking for, *is*—and we are someone who *has* it.

In Maria's case, she needed to keep her eyes open for the appearance of her new home; not just any home, but one that would meet her desire for safety and independence. This meant she should be looking in a better neighborhood, perhaps, and within her price range. Maybe a room-mate would be appropriate. She also needed to look for a home that would contribute to her sense of beauty and passion, sensuality, empowerment, accomplishment, and connectedness. OK, that's a lot, but it doesn't hurt to ask. On the contrary, *you have to ask*.

We have to be vigilant for the arrival of what we're asking for, because when it shows up, it is an opportunity that we should jump on. In Maria's case, when the home that fits her "wish list" shows up, in whatever deliciously miraculous way the Universe provides it, she should take it. Simple as that. You would be amazed how often we fail to receive what we ask for, only because we don't believe it when it comes. We don't recognize it, we question it, or we just think about it too much—and then the opportunity is gone. What is required here is detachment.

Detachment

Detachment means allowing the Universe to bring you what you ask for, in the way the Universe sees best. This will often look a lot different than what we are familiar with, but if we are too attached to having things show up looking the way we're used to, they will. They'll show up in exactly the way we're used to, which is based on our past experience, which is exactly what we are trying to move on from. Attachment to the familiar means we may miss what the Universe is offering us, something beyond the range of our experience, which may be more in alignment with our goals than we can even imagine.

Let me give you a personal example of this. When I finished my undergraduate studies at the university, and decided to go on to get my doctorate in chiropractic, I was your typical penniless college student. Having no money left for graduate school, I applied for grants and scholarships. I received enough money in grants to pay for one semester of chiropractic college, which is a ten-semester program; I had no idea how I would pay for the other nine semesters. Reluctant to take out the massive student loans that would be needed to get me through to a doctorate degree, I started my manifestation exercises, asking for a source of money that would pay for my education. I stated the reason behind this request in the simplest, most meaningful terms:

I wanted to get an education in order to bring healing and love to people, and to myself. I decided to take several months off after finishing my undergrad work, in order to work full-time and save up some money for chiropractic college, and I found a terrific job with great pay that I could continue part time after returning to school. It was close to the chiropractic college, so I rented my first very own (tiny, tiny) apartment nearby. I settled in, adopted a pair of kittens to keep me company, and was on my way... happy as a clam. Until I got fired from my terrific job.

I was devastated, partly because I had never been fired before, and I was really embarrassed; but also because I felt as if the universe had let me down. After all, I had done my spiritual homework. I wanted to spread healing, and love! What could be wrong with that? I looked and looked for a new job, but nothing seemed to come together for me. Finally, just as the first semester of chiropractic college was starting, and only to keep from being evicted, I took a crummy little waitressing job. I had saved exactly no money for my other 9 semesters.

It turns out the owner of the restaurant where I was now working had a silent partner, who would come to help wait on tables during the busy shifts on the weekends. While he wasn't actually very good at waiting on tables, he was tall and handsome, and extremely kind. That is what the Universe brought me. We were married at the end of my second semester, over 20 years ago now, and there has been a lot of healing and love in that time. And yes, he helped pay for my education.

The point here is that the universe provided me with exactly what I asked for, but in a way that I never could have planned myself. If I had been too attached to the "terrific job" as the answer to my manifestation requests, I might have given up and not started chiropractic college. The Universe's answer to my request for healing and love turned out to be much bigger and better than just a job.

DR. CORA B. LLERA, D.C.

Creation: the Ultimate Exercise in Choice

After I explained her manifestation "homework," I gave Maria the Wild Rose flower essence to take home and use with her manifestation exercises. She called a few days later to tell me that they seemed to be working.

Maria had just about lost her connection with her own life, her purpose and her passion. She needed to be reminded why she came here, to this tumultuous world of duality and physicality, and renew her commitment to that. The gypsy had lost her colors, had become faded and bitter, old and lost. Maria realized that her own "color" was her gift, and to lose her belief in the value of that gift was to lose not only her passion for life, but also her ability to help others renew their own passion for life. Depression is the inevitable result of this loss of passion, the loss of meaningful direction to our life.

When we define our direction and our goals in life in terms of need—need for financial security, need for attention and acclaim, etc.—life becomes a struggle, and frankly a rather tiresome one, that is focused around what we need in order to survive. Life becomes a battle to avoid death, and ironically, in the end we always fail. When we redefine our goals in terms of what we want: what we aspire to, and what inspires us—what we want to contribute, what we want to experience while we make that contribution and as a result of making it, what we want to have in order to make that contribution, and make it more, and better—the flow is completely different. Need is a linear flow from birth until death, a futile race against time. Want is circular, a seamless spiral of aspiration and fulfillment, inspiration, elevation and expansion. Need is based on fear of death. Want is based on love of life. You choose.

SIGNATURE ENERGY WORK

* * * * * * * * *

The examples of Sam and Maria demonstrate just a few of the techniques that can be employed to transform energy. They also illustrate the fact that a clear picture of the signature energy of the core question, and its answer, is helpful in the energy-work process. This clear picture comes from assembling the pieces that I have found in the SEWLINE, and interpreting them as a whole. Interpreting. Yes, that is a subjective skill, an artform, really. And as with any artform, you must first familiarize yourself with your instrument by understanding each of its parts, mastering the technical skills involved. Then, after a lot of practice, you can forget about all that and just *play*. The beauty of Signature Energy Work is that the work *is* the play.

So now I'd like to revisit some of the specific qualities of energy found in our SEWLINE to gain a more thorough understanding of how to play with the energy: how to put together an energy-work session that will move and transform the energy of our core question.

CHAPTER 8

WORKING THE LEVELS

Energy moves best when we use energy of comparable qualities to move it. In Case Study #2, we worked on the physical energy of Sam's "block" using physical energy in the form of deep massage and adjustment. We brought in the emotional energy that had been blocked using feelings of nurturing and maternal love. In the case of Maria, we used spiritual (angelic) energy to move a spiritual pattern (her "Wild Rose") out of her heart chakra. Let's look at working with the different qualities of energy by first focusing on each of the respective levels of the signature energy field.

PHYSICAL LEVEL

If my patient presents with some kind of physical complaint, I can be sure that it will require some type of physical energy work to move it. Depending on the location, excess physical energy can present in many forms, ranging from inflammation, to muscle spasm, to tumor. Deficient physical energy can present as fatigue, weakness, cold, numbness, etc. Some conventional medical diagnostic procedures may be appropriate to monitor these types of symptoms. If the energy turns out to be something pathological, for example a cyst, a referral to a medical doctor is definitely in order. This does not mean that the energy couldn't also be treated with Signature Energy Work; on the contrary, I think it's all the more needed in the case of pathology; however, the physical aspect of the energy should be monitored by an appropriate professional.

There are many ways to approach moving physical energy, depending on its qualities, but here are some suggestions:

Massage (Rolfing, Neuromuscular therapy, etc.)
Chiropractic adjustment or Osteopathic manipulation
Craniosacral therapy
Movement (stretching, exercise, Trager, Feldenkreis, Tai Chi, etc.)
Acupuncture/acupressure
Heat/Ice
Magnetic Therapy
Herbal Medicine
Nutritional supplements

EMOTIONAL LEVEL:

When the energy to be worked is related to the emotional level, it means we need to change an emotional pattern, a habitual pattern of emotional reaction. Emotional energy will be needed in the energy work; the patient needs to invest his feelings into the energy work process.

If the energy is to be moved **out** of the area, we need to access and clear the submerged, stored emotions. Recall that accessing emotional energy patterns can be done in two ways: directly or indirectly. In the direct method, the patient focuses her attention directly on the emotional energy pattern, observing it fully from a neutral, nonjudgmental state of mind. Ancient Taoist philosophy calls this the middle way, the state of centeredness from which we can surrender the idea that something is positive or negative, and see it as it is, without judgment. The middle way requires development of something called the "witness": what in Eastern philosophies is known as *samadhi*, or in Judeo-Christian philosophy would be called *the peace which passeth all understanding*. Leslie Temple-Thurston, in her book *The Marriage* *of Spirit*, gives some wonderful exercises on developing the witness. She explains that a part of us is always vigilantly observing ourselves: noting our emotional reactions, our irrational and dysfunctional behaviors, etc. Once we notice that witnessing part of ourselves, we can take steps to cultivate it; make it stronger and more productive. It may be helpful to go back to the moment in time when the emotional pattern involved became set in the body, as Nancy did when she focused on her "nose job." This time, however, we can experience the emotions from the point of view of the neutral witness. As the patient re-experiences the emotion in a more detached manner, she can complete the process that was started back when the emotion originally occurred; she can observe what happened to her from a bird's eye view, removed from the original circumstances that seemed so threatening at the time, and from this, more centered, vantage point, she can fully process the emotions – she can let the energy of the emotions pass through her.

The emotions were too powerful, back at the original moment of trauma or shock. It wasn't safe, under those circumstances, to experience them fully. But in viewing those same circumstances again, from the perspective of the neutral observer—who, merely by virtue of the fact that she is now observing, knows that she will survive the circumstances—it becomes possible to feel the full range of these emotions; to allow them to pass fully through without stopping them when they become scary or messy, and to come out on the other side of them. When we emerge from this experience intact, we gain the knowledge that negative emotions are painful, but they don't have to be dangerous. Their danger is only an illusion. This knowledge breeds compassion: for ourselves when we are feeling strong emotions, and for others when they are traveling through emotionally difficult passages. This is the compassion that comes from experience, also known as wisdom.

Emotional release is a very important and delicate process. If you don't feel comfortable or qualified to handle an emotional patient, it's very appropriate to refer them to a qualified therapist. But I must warn you that when you create a safe and relaxing environment for someone, he may feel comfortable enough to release emotions spontaneously, without any help or formal permission. You should at least be ready, and know what you want to do if this happens. Usually there is nothing you need to do except to let the person emote, while conveying to him in supportive words or with a gentle touch, or even just a look, that he's OK and that you are OK with his emotions. Obviously, telling the patient not to be emotional in your presence is about the worst thing you could do, so if that's how you feel, DON'T DO THIS WORK WITH OTHERS.

When we can allow ourselves to fully feel the emotion – the sadness, the anger, the loss—it can run its course, and then it naturally dissipates. I liken it to a thunderstorm; lots of ominous clouds and wind, then thunder and lightning, then tremendous drenching rain. And then it's over. The sun comes out, and life goes on. When I find a patient who repeatedly tests for emotional energies that I can't get them to access, meaning that they are unable or unwilling to feel the emotions involved, then I know I need to refer them for professional psychotherapy. This happens often, and it's good to put my patient into the hands of someone with the skills and training to specialize in creating a safe environment, and establishing the kind of deep rapport with the patient that fosters emotional processing.

If the emotional energy is to be moved *in* to the patient's body, rather than out, then the nature of the emotion must be noted—joy, encouragement, satisfaction, etc.—and then experienced fully at a feeling level by the patient, as it is allowed to move in. This was the case with my patient Sam, who needed to move the emotional energy of Mother—nurturing, safety, love—in to his body.

There are many indirect techniques that facilitate the taking in and moving out of emotional energy in the body. Here are a few:
Breathwork
Music
Drumming
Flower essences and homeopathic remedies
Massage and emotional-release oriented bodywork
Acupuncture/Acupressure
Movement

Direct techniques for accessing emotional energy might include:
Dialogue
Role Playing
Writing/Journaling
Meditation

MENTAL LEVEL:
If the energy to be moved is of the mental level, then we will be shifting the patient's habitual thought patterns: his ideas, and beliefs. I can't do this for the patient, or to the patient; I can only assist them in doing it themselves. Any indirect technique can act as a catalyst, but a direct technique—such as hypnotherapy, meditation, or visualization—must be added in order to bring the unconscious beliefs into conscious focus, and allow the patient to intentionally revise these mental patterns according to a more self-aware choice. Muscle-testing is very useful in finding the exact nature of unconscious beliefs. A belief pattern that is causing a problem is usually either extremely obsolete, or it's contradictory by its very nature; it is always limiting the patient's ability to grow.

Putting these beliefs into words in a conscious way is often all it takes to transcend them, but it reinforces the transformation to choose a suitable replacement belief, and to let the body know that this is the new norm.

To illustrate this point, let me tell you about Cathy.

CASE STUDY #6 - CATHY

Cathy presented in my office with acute, severe lower back pain, which had first started about two weeks prior. At that time she sought deep-tissue massage therapy to treat the problem. Her massage therapist had focused mainly on the ilio-psoas muscles, which attach to the front of the lower spine and connect to the front of the hips. Cathy explained that this therapy had helped her enormously, giving her nearly complete relief. The pain had returned, however, two days before she came to see me.

Muscle-testing indicated that the problem was related to the mental level, and was located in the gallbladder as well as the large intestine. Energy was required to be moved *in* to both organs, energy represented qualitatively by the flower essence Vervain. The *Flower Essence Repertory* describes Vervain as follows:

> *Vervain soul types naturally possess strong forces of passionate idealism. They give themselves fully and completely to the work or cause in which they believe. However, they can become so convinced of the rightness and urgency of their beliefs that their natural charismatic capacities degenerate into those of the zealot or fanatic. Their true leadership ability is afflicted, for the Vervain type's incredible intensity can overwhelm and prevent others from making their own energetic connection to the project or cause which is being promoted. Such an individual can be characterized as possessing not only great intensity but also great physical tension, which results in many nervous and digestive problems, and in extreme cases may lead to nervous breakdown.*

These persons are usually unaware of their true energy levels, and often push their bodies completely beyond their natural capacities. In fact, there is very little connection to the physical body or to the physical world, because this type lives so fervently in the world of ideas and ideals. Vervain is particularly an embodiment remedy, helping the soul to center and ground its tremendous enthusiasm. In this way, the body becomes a natural regulator and harmonizer for the abundant spiritual forces which pour out of such a person. When the fiery light of Vervain radiates through the medium of the body and the physical world, it becomes more luminous and contained. Such soul ardor is able to inspire, lead, and heal others.

When two locations test positive, as with Cathy, I have to go back and test to see if there is one of the two that should be treated first. With Cathy, it was the gall bladder. The gall bladder is the organ whose physiological function is to store and deliver the bile to the digestive tract. The old-fashioned term for bile is "gall". Hence the name. Gall is a term that connotes courage, assertiveness, or "chutzpah". I look at the mental aspect of the gall bladder as being related to decisiveness. Having the "gall" to make a difficult decision. It would seem that Cathy needed some of this, but in a regulated, harmonized, Vervain kind of way. I put a few drops of Vervain on my hands, and gently worked the gall bladder reflex area in the abdomen. As I worked, I asked her what was the decision that she was working on in her life. She said two things came to mind. First was regarding her work, and wanting to move out of her current job, to become self-employed. Cathy explained that she is licensed and trained as a nurse-practitioner, but because she was currently working in a dermatology office, she felt her skills were extremely under-utilized, as well as under-appreciated. She felt that she had much more to offer, and wanted to open her own practice. To go out "on her own".

The second thing that came to mind was that Cathy might be releasing some religious/spiritual issues from her past. This sounded to me like a large-intestine pattern. The large intestine, as I discussed back in Chapter 6, is the organ that is in charge of storing and releasing waste products from the digestive tract. Mentally, the large intestine is responsible for storing and releasing old ideas and beliefs. All in all, I explained to Cathy, it's about letting go of old shit. In all the senses of the word.

I moved my hands down into the lower abdomen, bringing the Vervain energy into the large intestine reflex area, and questioned Cathy about the religious and spiritual issues that she felt needed to be released. The large intestine points sit in the middle of the ilio-psoas muscles, and they felt tight and congested under my hands. Cathy paused for a minute, taking long slow breathes to help herself relax into the pain I was causing by stirring up these points. It seemed to me that she was also considering how much she wanted to reveal to me on this subject. After all, she came to treat her back pain, and here we were talking excrement and spirituality, all at the same time. Considerable subjects.

She revealed that she had been feeling very upset in the past couple of weeks about the continuous stream of stories in the news concerning abuse of young people by Catholic priests. She explained that she had gone to Catholic schools as a child, and felt that she had been physically, mentally, emotionally and spiritually abused by the nuns who were her teachers. They would punish her physically by hitting her with a paddle over her lower back and buttocks area, while telling her things like, "You're a sinner."

"You'll never come to any good in your life."

"You're a little slut who men will use and then cast aside."

"The only place you'll end up is in a home for unwed mothers."

She had vivid memories of being told these things repeatedly. She was just 9 years old at the time, she explained, and so innocent that she still played with dolls. She didn't really understand what they meant—she was too naïve—but she understood the paddle.

She would go home from school and cry to her mother that the nuns were hitting her. Her mother would respond by telling her that, "If the nuns hit you, you must have done something to deserve it."

Even one day when my mother came into my bedroom while I was dressing, and saw the rainbow of different colored bruises from my back down to my knees, she still sent me back to school. With the nuns. Every day. Except of course the two times I got to miss school because I was in the hospital. Being treated for my injuries. The message from my mother was clearly, "You're on your own."

Ah. Interesting choice of words. Being "on her own," in Cathy's subconscious files, was not at all a good thing. It was a very scary and dangerous thing. And, from the way she described it, painfully intertwined with the negative Vervain energy—overzealous righteousness—of the nuns. This was clearly the religious/ spiritual issue that she had mentioned needed to be released. In addition, her belief that being "on her own" was unsafe, needed to be transformed by the positive, harmonizing energy of Vervain.

As the large intestine points opened up and relaxed, I could feel the area coming to balance. I retested to see if the gall bladder and large intestine were complete. This tested positive, so I checked to see if any other locations needed attention. This too tested positive, so I started my locating questions again from the beginning. The second chakra showed up as needing energy input. No other qualifiers for the energy tested, so I just set my intention to move light into the field there. As I did this, I felt intuitively that

Cathy needed to experience drawing the light in to the second chakra herself, but specifically light energy in the form of Goddess/Mother—a pure, unconditional, feminine God-energy that was just for her, and that she could draw on at any time. I asked her to focus on this, drawing the Feminine energy into her second chakra as she inhaled, and pushing it up toward her heart as she exhaled. With each breath, the channel of energy flow from her second chakra to her heart chakra opened and cleared, and the reservoir of Feminine energy in her heart chakra expanded. As she continued, her entire field opened up, lightened, and relaxed.

Eventually I asked her to reverse the flow and radiate the Goddess/Mother energy outward from the second chakra, toward her 9-year-old self; filling and surrounding her with the energy. As she breathed into this, I told her to notice how she could, at will, radiate this same energy toward her clients. She could do this any time, on her own. She nodded blissfully.

I finished the session by working some muscular trigger points in the lower back area and around the pelvis, at the same time pointing out to Cathy that it was time to let go of the belief that "on her own" was necessarily something that would lead her to pain and humiliation. In light of the presence and accessibility of this powerful, loving Feminine energy, could she see now that being on her own merely meant that there was no need for any intermediary between herself and her Source? She could let go of the belief that the nuns, the Church, and even her own mother had to stand between her and the feminine face of God, and do her work from a place of connecting directly with God, on her own.

I sealed this transformation of mental energy into Cathy's physical body with an adjustment to the appropriate areas of her spine—those related to the gall bladder and large intestine—and gave Cathy a bottle of Vervain to take home and use for a couple of weeks. When I handed her the Vervain description from the *Flower Essence Repertory* to read, she mentioned that she had been having various digestive problems lately, and had already scheduled an appointment with an internist to run some tests. I agreed that diagnostic testing to rule out any serious pathology is always a good idea, and in addition, I suggested she might want to pursue some acupuncture treatments if the symptoms persisted. I stressed, however, that it was just as important that she follow up with some psychotherapy to address the childhood abuse issues that we had just looked at. When I explained that I thought this was one of the things that her body was trying to tell her, by giving her such acute back pain, she agreed to check into it.

SPIRITUAL LEVEL:

When we are working with energy that is of the spiritual layers, we are creating a change in the contexts, or underlying and connecting themes of our lives. At this level of work we are consciously accessing, examining and shifting our beliefs and assumptions about our purpose in life, and about the nature of Life itself. This is powerful work - a task that must be approached with a very calm, centered spiritual focus on the part of the practitioner. This focus takes preparation to create, and practice to maintain. Let me say it more clearly; doing Signature Energy Work on a regular basis is something that requires a certain amount of self-maintenance. That said, however, I believe that I won't be called on (by my muscle-testing) to work at the spiritual level if I am not ready to go there.

As I go, I am assisting my patient in accessing the spiritual level of his signature energy field, but I am also being offered an opportunity to access the spiritual level of my own signature energy, which means expanding my conscious awareness beyond its normal everyday boundaries. In order to sustain this level of expansion and connection, while at the same time being fully present to the patient's energy, I must be fully grounded:

consciously connected to my own physical body and my physical surroundings (see Appendix E: Grounding and Connecting).

Before beginning, I ask if I am sufficiently "grounded and connected" to proceed in moving the energy at hand. I then ask if I need any assistance. I often get a "yes" response to this question, which lets me know that I need to invoke the presence of spiritual helpers to handle the job. I can then proceed to ask what, or who, on the spiritual plane is going to be helping me, or I can ask for one of my spiritual guides or helpers to be present to assist me. Often, however, I merely make a general request for "guidance, healing, and protection from our guides, teachers, and friends in the light". If my patient is familiar with his own spiritual aspects, I will ask him to connect spiritually, and request his spirit guides to join the group.

If spiritual energy is being moved *in* to the area, then I want to help draw the energy offered by my spirit and/or spirit helpers into the patient's body. After using the information that we have received, from the SEWLINE, to create as clear an understanding as possible of the nature of this energy, we are then ready to draw the energy in to the patient's signature energy field. I like to use my breath in this process: drawing the spirit energy into my own signature energy field as I inhale, and focusing on pushing it out of my field (usually, but not always, through my hands) into the area in question on the patient's body. I can ask the patient to do the same; drawing in the spirit energy—and the new spiritual understanding that it carries—from his higher self or guides with the inhale, and pushing it into the involved area of his body on the exhale. This effectively inundates the area with spiritual energy. Let me illustrate with the example of Sylvia.

CASE STUDY #7 - SYLVIA

Sylvia is a teacher of physical education, so she has a very physical job. This prompts her to come in fairly regularly for chiropractic adjustments and energy work, and she came in on this particular day complaining mostly of fatigue. Sylvia is the type of person who generally delights in causing fatigue in others, so I questioned this complaint. She confessed that she had been feeling unusually stressed lately, since giving notice at her job that she would be leaving at the end of the school year. She laughed at herself, saying that you would think having quit her job would make her feel less stressed, rather than more. She realized, however, that although she had a long list of interesting projects, which she had been wanting to take on for years and never had the time for, she was feeling uneasy about the lack of structure—and the excess of unknown—that was now looming in front of her. She was, frankly, scared about moving into this new phase of her life.

I muscle-tested Sylvia, asking what we needed to know about her fatigue. The spiritual level was indicated, and the chakras. But in this case each of the classic seven chakras tested negative, meaning that the answer was to be found in a chakra, but not in chakras 1-7. I proceeded to test farther "up": the eighth chakra, again negative, then the ninth, positive. The ninth chakra needed energy to be moved *in*, and there was a block in place preventing this. The block tested negative for any qualifying information, and the energy to be moved *in* tested positive for WHAT as well as WHERE. The WHAT turned out to be related to two flower remedies: Pink Monkeyflower and Forget-Me-Not. The WHERE showed as another chakra, the third.

I explained to Sylvia that the ninth chakra is the threshold to the spiritual layer. It is something like a multi-dimensional, permeable membrane that surrounds us like a shell, and is itself surrounded by the spiritual energies that connect us to our Higher Self. In order to bring this spiritual energy from the ninth chakra into the body, then, we need to channel it through a portal: one of the lower seven chakras, in this case the third chakra. I pointed out that while Sylvia has obviously been blocking the influx of this ninth chakra energy, it was apparently not necessary for us to go into the details of why or how she was blocking; probably because there's nothing about that she didn't already know.

Sylvia rolled her eyes and grimaced in agreement, adding that she had been experiencing a vague sense of tightness and pain in her stomach area lately, but hadn't really thought too much about it, until now.

I consulted the *Flower Essence Repertory*, to understand the nature of the spiritual energy that we were going to be moving.

PINK MONKEYFLOWER: *Pink Monkeyflower treats a type of fear which resides in the deepest recesses of the soul: the fear of being exposed, of seeing one's pain and vulnerability. Such persons experience a profound sense of shame, and thus have a need to hide or mask themselves as a form of protection. The Pink Monkeyflower type withdraws in a way that is more pronounced than ordinary shyness, for the soul is attempting to cover deeply internalized wounds from the past. Most frequently, early childhood trauma or abuse – or exploitative and debasing experiences at any phase in life – are the hidden factors in such behavior. These souls are highly sensitive and bear deep pain within themselves. They very much want to reach out and be loved by others, but often fail at making real contact. Such individuals are highly sensitive to being seen, both literally and metaphorically. They are also very vulnerable to being touched and making physical contact with others. Pink Monkeyflower gently opens such souls by helping them to take emotional risks again. In this way, they begin to experience the love and the contact which they so desperately need and want. Pink Monkeyflower is a remedy which is especially effective for the heart, teaching that it is only by remaining open and risking vulnerability that one can experience the warmth of human love and affection.*

FORGET-ME-NOT: If we are to heal the wounds imposed on human culture by its overly materialistic viewpoint, it is necessary to lift our consciousness of the human family to include those souls who live outside the earthly dimension. Our hearts can naturally feel grief and concern for a living child who is abandoned and lacks the loving care and attention of a family; however, our materialistic bias makes us totally oblivious to the needs of souls who have departed from the physical realm. This blindness prevents us from providing sustenance and support to such souls, and also from receiving guidance and counsel from them for our earthly affairs. Yet establishing healthy contact with souls beyond the physical dimension is not easy. Many attempt unlawful contact through lower astral currents using drugs, sexuality, mediumism, or dangerous occult techniques. Rather than using these methods, we must be able to make contact with such souls in a heartfelt, conscious manner. The path of soul communion beyond the earthly threshold is a path of love – it depends on our ability to believe in the continued existence of the soul who has departed from physical form; remaining faithful to, and continuing to nurture the bonds of love which began on Earth. Forget–Me-Not helps awaken the soul to this higher level of heart exchange. It is an important essence to consider following the initial stage of grief after the death of a loved one, and can be very helpful for those who have never fully resolved their feelings of isolation and abandonment following the loss of an important family member or friend during childhood. Forget-Me-Not can also be used by expectant parents who wish to establish a conscious link with the soul seeking to be incarnated through them, or it can be beneficial when one wishes to understand the deeper, karmic soul connection which inspires or challenges any current relationship. In all these instances, Forget-Me-Not guides us toward greater love for the human family, and greater awareness of the incredible depth, beauty, and possibility of soul-based relationships.

This is a lot of information, and I wondered how to relate it to Sylvia's ninth chakra/third chakra pattern, as well as to her history and personality, at least what I knew of it. I felt as if I was looking at a jumbled collection of intricate puzzle pieces, and it was my job to decide how to put them together. Once again, I knew that engaging my intuition would be required, so with that in mind I took a deep, centering breath, and tried to consider the facts from a relaxed state, allowing my thoughts to percolate. In situations like these I know that there is not just one, single, right answer. The puzzle can be assembled into many forms, and each has value, so the secret is to just engage the subjective self, and see what shows up. First, I knew that Sylvia's reason for quitting her job was that she had developed a very specialized program of body awareness training that she had been teaching to private clients for some time now. She was preparing to teach independently, away from the barriers that a formal educational institution placed between herself and her students. This would allow her creativity to be uncensored and more fully appreciated, but barriers work two ways. Escaping the rigidity of the school's curriculum would also mean losing the security and relative anonymity that the school's structured atmosphere provided. She would be exposed, both professionally and emotionally: professionally, because she could no longer hide behind the mask of "gym teacher"—she would become known for her own work, and she would become known by name; emotionally, because she could no longer use her professional persona as a buffer between herself and the emotional life of her students. As soon as she let go of such artificial structures as curriculum, classroom time constraints, semesters, exams, and graduation, she would be left with just herself, her work, and the bond that the work makes between herself and the student. Her work would become much more private, in all the senses of the word. It would become intimate.

Second, it was interesting that the ninth chakra energy was to be moved into Sylvia's body through the third chakra. The third chakra is the power chakra; the energetic center that processes our beliefs and feelings about our own personal power, and how we wield that power. Both Pink Monkeyflower and Forget-Me-Not are heart-oriented remedies, and yet their energies are moving from Sylvia's ninth chakra—her Higher Self, her Spirit—into her third chakra. This would indicate to me that the positive qualities of these remedies—emotional openness and courage, awareness of and connection to the spiritual levels—*are* her power, but had been held in storage in the ninth chakra, as yet unwielded.

Third, it seemed that Sylvia was now ready to take her power out of storage, and the way to do that was by opening to her ninth chakra, the doorway to her own Higher Self, for guidance and direction. The flower remedies were, again, a clue about how to access her spiritual self: through her emotions and her spiritual awareness. The fact that this access had been blocked, but that we got no more information about the block, told me that Sylvia had been *purposely* blocking her emotions and her spiritual awareness. This blocking may have been an appropriate survival mechanism for the academic setting, where emotions and spiritual connection are not highly valued. The possibility for expansion into unexplored territory, to be provided by the intimate setting of private teaching, however, had now turned the protective block into an impediment; it had to go.

I placed my hands over Sylvia's third chakra, and allowed my fingers to sink in deeply, finding the point of resistance in the abdominal muscles that protect the area. I asked Sylvia to breath fully into my hands, drawing the spiritual energy that surrounds her into the third chakra, funneling it into the area of resistance and melting the block, allowing the spiritual energy to fill the chakra.

SIGNATURE ENERGY WORK

We worked this way for several minutes, until I could feel Sylvia relax. Her breathing became deeper, unrestricted and rhythmic. At this point I asked her to open up to the guidance of her spiritual self—to allow her Higher Self to provide her with pictures or words or, most importantly, feelings that would show her where she is heading in her work, and in her next phase of life.

I asked Sylvia also to indicate to me when she had gotten the information she needed: when it was complete. I waited, allowing the images and feelings to flow in through my own intuitive "eye," until Sylvia nodded softly. This done, I adjusted her spine in the areas neurologically related to the third chakra, to release the physical energy of the block. I gave her some Pink Monkeyflower and some Forget-Me-Not to take home and use, reminding her that she needed to form a new habit of checking in with her emotions and her "ninth-chakra-self" regularly for guidance; to teach herself to trust, rather than to block.

If I am moving spiritual energy *out* of an area, as I did with Maria in Chapter 7, I want to choose a method that I'm comfortable with. There are many methods related to spiritual energy release available, and this is a whole course of study on its own, but the important thing is to be prepared. When I am moving spiritual energy out of someone's signature energy field, I am dealing with energy that doesn't belong where it is. This often means that the energy is not very balanced, clean, or even friendly, for that matter. I don't get involved here unless I feel really confident that I know what I'm doing. There are many wonderful practitioners, of all sorts, who specialize in just this kind of work, so I am not afraid to acknowledge my own limits, and refer appropriately.

That said, I use two basic methods for releasing spiritual energy. The first is to move the energy out of the patient's body and into my own field, and from there, offer it up to *my* spirit helpers to dispose of. This method requires rigorous attention to my own spiritual connection, as well as to my own spiritual cleansing procedures. Sometimes I prefer not to be such a literal intermediary for the energies, and use something a little more indirect. I can bring in spiritual energy from outside—in Maria's case I invoked Archangel Michael and his crew, often I will call in the patient's own spirit helpers—to envelop the energy in question and then move it out. It doesn't have to be this dramatic; frequently I can just move spiritual energy into the patient's body through my hands, as mentioned above, allowing that energy to surround the questionable energy and essentially "light-blast" it out of the patient's body.

Both Maria and Sylvia illustrate the importance of incorporating direct/internal techniques into the healing session. I could move the spiritual energies involved with the patient's problems myself, thus creating a change in her signature energy field that she would palpably feel, and allowing her to function more comfortably and freely. By engaging the patient into the process, however, and encouraging her awareness and understanding of the spiritual energies involved, she can create a shift in her spiritual understanding of *herself*. This elevated self-awareness is what prevents her from re-creating the problem. It's what allows her to grow.

CHAPTER 9

WORKING THE SIX W'S

Next, let me elaborate on working with some of the other qualities of energy, by looking at what I call the Six W's.

The "WHAT" Qualities:

Colors

The use of color in healing is an entire field of study unto itself, and one that has a long history. Light therapy, Colorpuncture, PUVA therapy, Ocular Light Therapy, Syntonic Optometry, Spectro-Chrome, color reflexology, and pranic healing, are just some of the color healing methods currently in use. Color healing is based on extensive scientific research, as well as ancient esoteric teachings, and I encourage you to research these healing techniques if you are interested in the power of color. For the purposes of this book, let's just cover the basic use of color in the context of Signature Energy Work. If color tests positive as a quality of the energy of my problem/question, it is an indication that I need to take color into consideration, both in my examination of the nature of the energy pattern of my core answer, but also in my energy-moving process. I can add color to my energy-moving techniques by placing an appropriately colored stone or lens directly on the body, over the location found during the SEWLINE testing, or simply by focusing my intention on moving a specific color of energy *in* or *out* of that area (as tested) during the energy-moving process. Below is a list of some of the attributes of the more common colors, taken from the writings of various experts:

Angeles Arrien, Ph.D., a cultural anthropologist who studied the meaning of colors from a cross-cultural perspective; Dinshah Ghadiali, a color therapy researcher from India who, in the early 1900's, studied the physiological effects of color on the human body; Stephen Co, a Master Pranic Healer; and Barbara Brennan, who uses color in her own energetic healing practice.

RED: Red is associated with love and desire, the development of trust for one's own feelings. It can also connote anger. Red stimulates the sensory nervous system, liver function, red-blood-cell production, and excretion of toxins. It is generally warming and stimulating to the Signature Energy field.

ORANGE: Orange is associated with vitality, ambition, and spontaneity. It accelerates regeneration of lung tissue, stimulates the thyroid gland, and inhibits the parathyroid gland. Orange is generally expulsive and cleansing, and can be stimulating to the immune system as well as to sexual potency.

YELLOW: Yellow is cross-culturally viewed as the human representation for light, and as such suggests spirituality or higher mental activity. It stimulates the neuromuscular system, the lymphatic system, and the digestive tract. Yellow is generally used for triggering tissue growth and repair.

GREEN: Green is associated with creativity and fertility, healing and nurturing. It equilibrates and balances the function and regeneration of all tissues, but especially endocrine tissues, and the tissues associated with the heart. Green is disinfecting and decongesting, and is often used for overall healing.

BLUE: Blue is seen cross-culturally as the color that represents wisdom and clarity, as well as emotionality. Blue is stimulating to the pineal gland, but calming to the nervous system. It is generally used to slow or inhibit energy movement, and to reduce inflammation or energetic excess.

INDIGO: Indigo is associated with a deep connection to the spiritual levels, intuition, and devotion. It stimulates parathyroid gland function, inhibits thyroid function, and increases white-blood-cell levels.

VIOLET: Violet is associated with leadership and self-respect. It is stimulating to the spleen, and inhibiting to the pancreas and muscle tissues. Violet is generally used for clearing low-frequency energy, and magnifying higher-frequency energy.

GOLD: Gold is associated with wisdom, grace, and cosmic consciousness. It is generally used to energize the field, especially at the spiritual levels.

SILVER: Silver is associated with communication and purification, and creates a powerful purging effect on the Signature Energy field.

Flower Essences

Flower essences were developed for use as a treatment modality by Dr. Edward Bach, an English bacteriologist, in the early 1900's. In spite of the fact that flower essences have been in use for nearly a century, an exact scientific explanation as to how they work has been difficult to find. Most of the research on flower essences has been carried out at the psychic and intuitive, rather than objective levels, perhaps because flower essences seem to have a much more powerful effect on the subtle anatomy than on the physical body. Bach believed flower essences work mainly on the spiritual levels. While I really love flower essences as tools for directly accessing and understanding the energy of the core answer, they are also a very effective adjunct to Signature Energy Work when used in an indirect manner: by prescribing flower essences as a treatment, according to the traditional homeopathic model, or by adding them to the energy-work process by applying to my hands a few drops of the flower essence that has shown up in SEWLINE testing. The flower essence then acts as a filter, imbuing the energy with the characteristics of the flower as the energy is moved.

One of my favorite "flower stories" is Dylan, so indulge me while I relate it to you.

CASE STUDY #8 - DYLAN

Dylan was three years old when I first saw him. His mother called me to make an appointment because Dylan had been experiencing chronic sinus-type symptoms—runny nose, headache, fatigue—for approximately the past 3 months. The family doctor had diagnosed Dylan with allergies, and had recommended that he be taken for a series of injections. This was not Dylan's favorite idea.

It is not uncommon for mothers to bring their children in to be muscle-tested for specific allergies. While muscle-testing is certainly not as objective as scratch testing, or blood testing, it is much less invasive, and can be remarkably accurate. I tested Dylan, using his mother as a surrogate, to determine what he might be allergic to. He tested weakly positive for melon and cat hair; so weakly, in fact, that I questioned whether they were really accountable for Dylan's symptoms. I asked if there was more that we needed to know about Dylan's allergies, and was led to the right lung and the liver. Both organs were being affected by the "allergy". I tested further, and found that the "allergen" was emotional in nature, rather than physical. This explained why the physical allergen—melon and cat hair—tested so equivocally. The "allergen" also tested as being represented by the flower essence Rock Water.

I explained my findings to Dylan's mother, telling her that the lung is the organ that processes the emotions of grief and loss, while the liver processes anger. I asked if Dylan had been exposed to any unusually large quantities of these emotions lately. Her eyes widened as she answered that her father-in-law, Dylan's grandfather, had died recently. Three months ago, to be exact, almost immediately before Dylan's sinus symptoms had begun. She went on to say that Dylan seemed to be taking his grandfather's passing quite well, and had been very tranquil in the questioning and answering that had gone on at home about death and dying. Dylan's older brother had been the one who seemed unusually sad and angry about losing his grandfather.

I handed Dylan's mom a copy of the *Flower Essence Repertory* explanation of Rock Water.

Rock Water, one of the original English remedies, is not made from a plant, but from the essence of a sacred, underground spring, where the Earth forces are concentrated and consecrated. Rock Water treats a condition of soul which is more mineral than plant-like; it is for those who have extremely rigid attitudes toward life. Although such souls have high philosophical ideals, they suffer from an inability to enjoy life, and their thoughts quickly crystallize into hardened dogma. They adopt schedules for work, or life patterns for eating and sleeping, which are overly restrictive and mechanical. If they are following a spiritual path, such individuals tend towards harsh asceticism, attempting to fit their lives into strict and narrow concepts of spiritual behavior. The essence of Rock Water helps such souls to develop more inner flexibility, and especially to feel the living, pulsing currents of their emotional life. In this way, such persons come more in touch with their feelings, which stream and flow from the inner being much as water courses from the Earth. This essence is sometimes indicated for those beginning flower essence therapy, or for those who cannot feel the results of flower essences. Rock Water opens the soul to the plant realm of consciousness, by helping it to experience the flowering, flowing qualities of the feeling life.

Dylan's mom smiled as she read the page, then looked up and said that this described her older son perfectly. It also described her late father-in-law. I told her, gently, that it seemed as if Dylan was allergic to his brother. Or at least to his brother's emotions. I explained that the normal procedure for food or environmental allergies is to completely eliminate exposure for a period of 90 days, and then gradually introduce the "allergen" to allow the body to accommodate it, if possible. I laughed, saying that this was obviously not a practical approach in this case. She responded that, coincidentally, since their grandfather's death, the boys had not only begun sharing a bedroom, but were sharing a bed. And nighttime seemed to be when Dylan's symptoms were the worst.

No wonder.

I suggested that perhaps in addition to treating both boys with Rock Water, Dylan's mom should think about changing the sleeping arrangements, at least for a while. I showed her where the lung and liver reflex points were on the body, and instructed her to put a few drops of Rock Water on her hands, and then rub them over these points, repeating the process about 4 times per day, if possible. In addition, I suggested that it might be helpful to both Dylan and his brother if she could spend some time with them each day talking about their feelings regarding their grandfather, and how to deal with those feelings—and negative feelings of any kind—perhaps through movement, coloring, storytelling, or just conversation. Dylan's mom was very happy to know that she could help both of her boys in such a tangible way, and left my office promising to use the Rock Water faithfully.

Later, she left a message on my voice mail, telling me that as she was driving home, she recalled that her husband's uncle, his late father's brother, also had chronic sinus problems since childhood, and had long ago lost his ability to taste food. It was just too coincidental that Dylan and his brother were repeating an emotional pattern that their grandfather and great-uncle lived with throughout their lives, but it was also great that we recognized the pattern, and found a way to work towards its resolution.

Traditional Homeopathic Remedies

Homeopathy was developed by Dr. Samuel Hahnemann, a German physician who, in the mid-1800's, came upon the principle of "like cures like", which refers to treating a sick patient by giving him a minute dose of the substance that, in a healthy person, would actually cause the same illness. This is similar to the concept of vaccination, where a small dose of a substance is administered in order to stimulate an immune response in the body. Homeopathy is primarily an energy healing modality, meaning that the effect of the homeopathic remedy does not follow the same physiological principles as a conventional medication. In general, homeopathic physicians prescribe homeopathic remedies after taking a very detailed history of the patient and his current illness, and then matching his symptoms with a list of the characteristics of specific remedies. Many of the traditional homeopathic remedies have interesting characteristics that can also be quite helpful in qualifying the nature of an energy pattern, in much the same way as the flower essences. I test for homeopathic remedies in the same way as for flowers, using funnel testing on a collection of remedies in order to single out the relevant one.

The "WHERE" Qualities:

The appearance of **WHERE** as a quality of the energy involved with our core question indicates that energy is going to, or coming from, somewhere specific. In terms of energy-work, this means that the energy is to be moved from one location to another. This was very much the case with Rafael.

CASE HISTORY #9 - RAFAEL
Rafael is a big guy, strong and athletic-looking, who is a gifted and highly trained massage therapist. He was working full time managing the books in his family's business, and only occasionally doing his massage work, when he came to me complaining of mid and upper back tension, as well as a sense of irritability and restlessness.

Muscle-testing on Rafael showed that all levels of the field were involved, and then took me to the hara[42] as my location. The SEWLINE results indicated that energy needed to be moved *out* of the hara, and then directed to (WHERE) the heart chakra, and then each chakra upward from there.

As I placed my hand on the hara, Rafael naturally slipped into a deep-breathing pattern, as though sucking in the energy through his hara in increasingly larger and more expansive breaths. His head gradually tipped back, his arms opening out away from his body like wings. I got a sense of the vastness of Rafael's capacity for drawing in and containing energy. As I moved my free hand up to his heart chakra, I could feel him pulling the energy naturally upward to fill it: putting the focus of his breath into the chakra, and then expanding his own energy into it. I realized, as I watched him, that he rarely allowed himself the luxury of unleashing the full measure of his own power into his heart. It was almost as if, for some reason, he had been keeping his power a secret, even from his own heart. Breaching the boundary of this secret created an explosive reunion of the energy of his personal power with the energy of love in his heart, like the meeting of two wild rivers. Having my hands on his heart chakra while it streamed with power was intensely expansive for my own energy field. I focused intently on my grounding, at the same time savoring the expansion, then moved my hands over the lung points and shifted my position to sit at his head. I braced myself, and placed my closed fist over the thymus area, where the extraordinary chakra called the "High Heart" is located. (The High Heart is considered an "extra" chakra that we, as humans, are developing as part of our spiritual evolution. For most of us, this chakra is mostly dormant. As I understand it, its function is to channel high spiritual energy directly to the heart—a vague definition, I know, but the extent of this chakra's purpose is not yet widely understood. Here again, my intuition gave me the hunch that bringing energy to Rafael's High Heart would be important.) Rafael's breath immediately quickened its pace, but was still so deep that rumbling waves of sound came out of him on each exhale. As the rhythm slowly ebbed, and his breath lengthened once again, while deepening even more, I opened my fist so that the full force of energy would move into the High Heart.

At that point, time stopped.

There was nothing but energy. Energy expanding. Energy flowing. Energy and breath, energy and breath, energy and breath.

It took everything I had to stay in my body against the crashing impact of that energy. Gradually, very gradually, the rush dissipated, and I could move my hands out to Rafael's upper back muscles to work the muscular trigger points there, releasing the resistance to the High Heart energy held in the muscles. I slowly made my way up into his neck and head, making sure that the fifth, sixth, and seventh chakras were open to receive the hara energy.

I spoke to Rafael afterward about how fully and naturally the energy moved through his body. I sensed this energy was a magnificent gift, but one that needed to be managed. He needed to learn how to navigate more consciously the flow of the energy, so that he could channel it comfortably and effectively as healing energy in his massage work. I suggested that he seek out someone with whom he could study Chi Gong, the ancient Chinese art of energy movement.

He hesitated at this. Taking in any kind of energy from anyone, he explained, was very difficult for him; he didn't have much trust for people's intentions, and felt very reluctant to place himself in the hands of a teacher who may not understand or respect him as a student. This certainly explained why Rafael's hara energy had been so disconnected from his heart. Distrust. Not only did he distrust his own power, he distrusted everyone else's power also.

Except mine, for some reason.

I have previously mentioned the phenomena of resonance; the resonance of the signature energies of the practitioner and the patient. I believe it was the resonance between my signature energy and Rafael's that allowed me to experience his energy so powerfully. The similarity of our respective energies, brought together, created a resonant combination that was greater than either of our energies alone. The nature of that similarity, then, warrants examination.

Much like Rafael, I have spent most of my life distrusting my power. I have spent decades, lifetimes more likely, looking for a source of power outside of myself, chasing around putting people and institutions and systems of knowledge on a continuous series of pedestals, only to have each one eventually fall off. The result has been an energetic armor around me made of disappointment, fear, and pain that both defends and restricts me. Distrust.

Perhaps it was the similarity of our energies that compelled Rafael to allow me to enter into his field and touch him, at so many levels. Certainly it caused me to be touched by his story, enough to take action and write the words you are reading now.

I suggested to Rafael that he should clearly express his intention to learn about how to manage his own energy, and direct this expression to the *Source* of his power, as he understood it. The Source would provide him the tools for that learning, perhaps in the form of a book, a class, or a trustworthy teacher. It doesn't really matter what form such information comes in, because each of us, alone, is the one who must integrate it into our being. Ultimately, we are always our own best teacher, and as such we attract to us exactly what we need in order to learn. We are all continually attracting exactly what we need to learn, but it's just so much quicker – and more pleasant - to attract intentionally, rather than by default.

I pointed out to Rafael that his capacity for holding and wielding energy was huge, and that if he didn't keep it moving, and maintain an appropriate outlet for it, it would eventually make him sick. He nodded in understanding, and then went on to explain that for the past few months, he and his wife had been living "temporarily" in a very small apartment, which they moved into while the new home that they recently purchased was being remodeled. He found himself squeezed into a space that was much too small for him, with none of his usual outlets for expression available to him; his musical instruments, his gardening tools, and his gourmet cooking utensils were all packed up in boxes, inaccessible. And of course the construction on the house had been delayed, repeatedly. He couldn't miss the parallel between his body, where all his power had been squeezed into the relatively tiny space of the hara, and his home. It was clear that the universe was trying to tell him that moving his energy was important, and that it was time to stop being afraid of his own power.

Amen to that.

The "WHO" Qualities:

The **WHO** qualities indicate that we need to move energy that is related to another person (or persons), in some form. If this energy is being moved *out* of the patient, it is often helpful to understand why the patient has been holding on to the energy, that is, why someone else's energy would be so resonant with the patient's. This allows the patient to transform that aspect of herself, thus eliminating the point of resonance with the "other's" energy. It may also be necessary to transform the nature of the other's energy, before sending it out. We saw this in the case of Maria, which demonstrates the fact that when we are moving non-human energy, special care—and sometimes special assistance—is needed to handle the energy, rather than just setting it loose as is, only to cause a problem somewhere else. When moving out human energy, we can transform the energy and then send it back to the person from whom it came. This way, we are performing a service not only for the patient, but also for the other person. An example of this is Diane.

CASE STUDY #10 - DIANE

Diane had been a patient of mine for quite a while, and was one of those rare patients who came prepared to do whatever kind of work was presented to her. From the very first day, she didn't even blink at the strange "trans-personal" places we would end up in during her sessions. This one was no exception.

Diane came in that day complaining of a persistent soreness in her left shoulder area since falling in her home approximately one week prior. She also showed me a nasty bruise, about twice the size of my hand, over her left hip, which was what she landed on when she fell. Without my prompting she went on to explain that at about the same time, she had come to a realization: In spite of a fairly continuous series of romantic relationships in her life, she had never actually had the experience of "making love". Her sexual encounters had always been just that, sexual only. She realized that, while she enjoyed sex, and found it very satisfying, she was missing the elements of tenderness and affection that went along with the experience of love within the sexual union. She had immediately brought this up to her boyfriend, who abruptly ended the relationship. Diane said that she actually felt a sense of relief about this, instead of her usual hysterical sadness when a breakup happened. The hip bruise was easily explained by the fall, and had, in fact, improved considerably in the past week. The shoulder, however, was not improving, and was not directly related to the mechanics of her fall. She wanted to know what the shoulder pain was trying to tell her.

Muscle testing showed that the pattern originated at the spiritual level, and the area of the body that held the answer to the question was the heart (ORGAN). The heart needed energy to be moved *out*. The energy to be moved out was related to a past life (WHEN), and was coming from a person other than herself (WHO).

I explained to Diane that we were going to be looking into a past life to find the answer, and she nodded agreement. She had experienced past life regression before, so she slid almost immediately into a deeply relaxed state on the table. I asked her to enter into the lifetime where she could get information about her shoulder pain, and waited, allowing the silence in the room to draw her attention away from her body on my table, and into the body in that other time and place.

Her eyes began to flicker back and forth rapidly under her closed eyelids, and a slow, contented smile came over her face. I watched a tear wander unattended down the side of her face, and then asked her what she perceived there, in that other self.

She spoke softly, saying she saw herself in another lifetime, living in a teepee.

We live by the river...a very natural place...someone is with me; I'm holding her in my arms. I love her. She's my wife...I'm a man. I feel such deep love for her, and such happiness in this place...I just want to hold her, and kiss her all of the time. Love and sex are not separated at all for us...so natural...it's all the same energy. It's an energy that connects us.

I instructed her to breath in some of that connecting, natural, love energy. To really take it in fully. This was obviously not the energy that needed to be moved out of her body; it seemed more like a gift, and an indication that we needed to continue in order to find the energy in question, but also a clue about its nature. I asked her to move forward, to the time when she lost this natural, loving energy; when she became separated from it.

Diane's countenance changed from day to night. Her body shrank with tension as she told me that she could feel herself in a completely different lifetime, this time as a woman. She had been abducted and dragged down into what looked like a dark, abandoned mining shaft by a man, who was now violently raping her. She could feel his energy invading her, and it was all about separation: The separation of his actions from any feeling, the separation of love and sex into two widely divergent streams. Diane seemed strangely calm as she described this to me. There was no terror or hysteria, but instead a distinct sadness. As though, after the beautiful energy she had just come out of in the "teepee" life, all she could feel for this rapist was sadness; pity.

I explained to Diane that it was this man's energy—the energy of rape, the energy of complete separation of love and sex—that needed to be moved out of her body. But first, I was going to ask her to do something very difficult. Difficult, but I knew she was up to the job. She nodded her willingness to proceed.

I asked Diane to look into the rapist's eyes, to connect her soul's energy to his.

No, I don't think I can see his eyes. All I can see is the light coming from the tunnel above us.

I let her know that I understood, but I persisted gently, asking if she could connect the energy of her heart to his heart, from the level of feeling instead of seeing. She nodded. I told her that I wanted her to give him a gift: the gift of that natural, loving energy from her teepee life where there had been no separation of love and sex. I asked her to begin by letting that beautiful energy fill her own heart, immersing any of the rapist's energy that was there with the love and connection she had felt there by the river; transforming, with her intention, the energy of separation into the energy of connection. This was easy for her, and she immediately began to breath deeply and relax into the same slow smile that I saw earlier. Then I instructed her to send his now-transformed energy outward from her heart to his, so that he could feel it in his own heart. So that he could have the experience of what connection felt like.

This touched her. The tears streamed down her face as she breathed deeper, pushing the breath out, smiling and crying all at once. Long minutes went by, as she breathed and I worked the muscles and reflex points around her heart. Finally she spoke, so softly that I had to ask her to repeat it.

I can see his eyes now...It's my grandfather. His eyes are my grandfather's eyes.

"Good," I said, "move that same energy now into your grandfather's eyes, into his heart. Give him the gift of that energy, because he really needs it." She sighed deeply, I think both in accordance with that statement as well as in determination to follow through.

I rounded out the treatment by adjusting the spinal points related to her heart, as well as adjusting the balance of her hips, to compensate for the bruising jar of her fall. I re-tested to make sure that we had completed the session, and to ask if there were any referrals or "homework" needed. What showed up was a flower remedy, Basil, for Diane to take and use as a follow-up to the treatment. Afterward Diane mentioned that she had always had a sense of "inappropriate" sexual energy coming from her grandfather when she was a child, and had often wondered, as an adult, if perhaps she had been sexually abused by him. She had no conscious memory of such, but she was sure that her own tendency to separate love from sexuality was at least partially due to the way sexuality was dealt with within her family culture, starting with her grandfather, who was the epitome of the macho patriarchal stereotype in which sex is used by men as a way to exert their power over women.

It was a new experience for Diane to look at her grandfather from an even more powerful vantage point: love. She now realized that the rapist in her past life, as well as her grandfather in this life, had never had one of the most fulfilling, joyful experiences that life has to offer; the integration of love and sexuality. From this point of view, she no longer felt fear or anger toward her grandfather/rapist, but rather a sense of compassion. She also felt a confident anticipation about re-creating that integration in her own, current life. She couldn't wait to get started on her next relationship, because now she knew exactly what she was looking for, and, more importantly, that her goal was not impossible. All she had to do was remember the sweetness of that lifetime by the river, and she knew that love, expressed through sexuality, exists.

Diane told me that her grandfather had died many years before, but she hoped that the energy she had sent him would be helpful to him, in his next life.

The *Flower Essence Repertory* describes Basil as follows:

The soul in need of Basil tends to polarize and separate the experience of spirituality and sexuality, believing that these cannot be integrated. This affliction is most evident in relationships where there is a compulsive need to seek sexual liaisons outside the main partnership. Quite often sexual activity is associated with that which is secret or sinful. There is also very strong attraction to pornography and other forms of illicit or illegal sexuality. The soul feels great tension between the polarities of spiritual purity and physical sexuality. In the unconscious struggle to reconcile these forces, the soul often capitulates to or becomes enmeshed in debasing and dehumanizing sexual activity. Basil flower essence helps the soul to experience the world and the Self as truly sacred and whole.

If the **WHO** energy that we are dealing with is to be moved *in* to the patient, this means we are drawing on energy that comes from someone else, and moving it into the patient's body. To facilitate this process, I usually have the patient visualize the other persons(s) involved, and allow their energy to flow in to the area in question. Such was the case with Sasha.

CASE STUDY #11 - SASHA

Sasha is one of the most gentle people I've ever met. She has a big family, and is a stay-at-home-Mom extraordinaire. She came to me complaining of stiffness in the left side of her neck that frequently extended into her left shoulder blade area. This had been persisting for months already by the time she saw me, and she had checked it out with her family doctor to make sure it was nothing serious. She was told that it was "stress related" and sent home with a prescription for muscle relaxers, which she found that she couldn't use, as they made her too woozy to function normally. She had called me after a detailed description of a signature energy work session by a friend from her religious community. She was wonderfully open to the idea that her problem might not be merely physical in origin, but may also have emotional, mental, or even spiritual components that needed to be addressed.

Muscle testing took me to Sasha's fifth chakra, the throat chakra, which needed energy moved **in** to it. This energy was related to (WHO) her husband, and was also related to the spiritual level of the signature energy field. In addition, there was a block in place, which prevented this energy from moving in. The block was related to the flower essence Oregon Grape, and was also spiritual in nature.

I explained this carefully to Sasha, keeping in mind the fact that she is a person who is very devoted to her religion, and wanting to make sure my concepts were presented in language that was accessible for her. Essentially, her husband's spirit, his Higher Self if you will, wanted to bring energy to her throat chakra, which is her center for communication, as well as her sense of truth. Her own spirit, or Higher Self, was blocking this energy for some reason—a reason that probably had something to do with the pattern of Oregon Grape. I read Sasha the description of Oregon Grape.

> *To trust in the goodness of others is to be nourished by the milk of human kindness. Regrettably, many souls are malnourished; they are unable to receive the sustaining love of others. Oregon Grape is indicated for those persons who are filled with paranoia; they see the world and those around them as hostile and unfair. These patterns were learned in childhood from the family or culture, and have not been healed; instead they fester in the soul and go on to infect all human relationships and social situations. Unfortunately, the soul who is gripped by this paranoid state creates the very reality he/she projects, for those who are treated in a hostile or mistrustful manner usually respond with an equal measure in return. Oregon Grape is widely applicable, but is especially indicated for the tension and ill-will which predominates in many urban environments. Through Oregon Grape the soul learns to break the basic pattern of mistrust. It realizes that it can look instead for the positive intentions of others, and create situations which generate good will and loving inclusion.*

Sasha and I agreed that the operative word here was mistrust. This was the energy of the block that her own Spirit had placed around her throat chakra. I acknowledged that it seemed odd that one's Spirit would do that; after all, mistrust is not what I would normally think of as being part of one's spiritual path. But Sasha smiled, and explained that in her religion, spiritual study is done didactically, meaning that students sit face to face and study a sacred text together by explaining it to each other, examining it in detail and often arguing over its meaning. Sasha had done this for years with her children, her friends, her family. But never with her husband. Never.

She agreed that the feeling of mistrust was very familiar to her, in fact something she had grown up with in her family and religious culture. She often felt that she mistrusted God, or at least the God that was taught to her by her family and her religious community. She had a profound desire, a compulsion even, to experience God first hand: to discover the nature of God on her own, without the distraction of prayers and rituals and other people's explanations. It wasn't until just within the past couple of years that she had overcome her reluctance to be misunderstood by those in her religious community who thought that such a pursuit was inappropriate, or impossible.

So, I questioned, her mistrust of anyone else's God had pushed her toward finding her own God? Sasha agreed, and I realized why her Spirit had put the mistrust block around her throat. This block was preventing energy from moving into Sasha's throat chakra, the energetic center that holds and processes the energy of truth. Sasha's Spirit was blocking anyone else's truth from entering in until Sasha had found the strength to examine her own, internal truth.

I pointed out that apparently her Spirit thought she was ready to release that block, at least in the context of her husband's spiritual truth. Sasha explained that her husband had asked her repeatedly, implored her, to study with him during the early years of their marriage. But she had always refused because she felt that if she did that, she would lose her truth to his. He would devour her somehow, with his passionate understanding of God as he saw it. She knew that he was disappointed that she was unwilling to share such an important part of his world with him, but eventually he stopped asking her to discuss spiritual matters with him, and hadn't brought it up in years. She acknowledged that it had left something of a hole in their relationship.

I asked her to close her eyes and visualize her husband's spiritual energy, to see it as clearly as she could in her mind's eye.

I instructed her to look at the blocking energy in her throat chakra and then, using her breath, open up the block to allow only her husband's energy to flow into her throat. I asked her to let his energy interact with hers, and to notice the effect that it had. She said that his energy felt warm, and flowed in with a rush. It felt different from her own throat energy, but not uncomfortable. The two energies swirled together, and while they seemed to influence each other—his made hers warmer, and hers made his lighter—they didn't blend completely. Each one held its integrity enough to be recognized as separate, and yet they were together, sort of peacefully coexisting. Lovingly coexisting.

Sasha left my office with the intention to invite her husband to study with her soon. About an hour after she left, she called me to say that her neck felt much better, and to relate something remarkable that had happened. Not ten minutes after she left my office, her husband called her, very excited about a passage of spiritual material that he had just read, and wanting to talk to her about it. They talked at length, and she was delighted by how respectful he was of her opinion, as well as how close she felt to him while they were sharing these ideas. It wasn't until after she hung up the phone that she remembered our session, and just had to call me. We agreed that we must be a pretty good team, to have created a change so fast!

The "WHEN" Qualities:

These qualities point me to a particular moment in time, related to the energy in question. If we are dealing with a blocking energy, as in the case of Sam, this would be the period of time when the block was put into place. If I am working with energy to be moved *out* of the body, examining the time period when that energy originated, before moving it out, is what is indicated. This was the case with Carmen.

CASE STUDY #12 – CARMEN: Part I

Carmen had been suffering for two weeks with a nagging neck pain, which occasionally radiated into her right arm. Her daughter was a patient of mine, and didn't like to see her mother suffering, so brought her in to see me.

The pattern of Carmen's pain—radiculopathy—is a pretty classic presentation, and usually responds well to traditional chiropractic care. When I muscle tested Carmen, however, something interesting showed up. Carmen's pain was coming from the emotional level. The location that I was led to was in the bone, specifically the second cervical vertebra, C2. This vertebra is the second one from the top, in the upper neck, and not the one that is usually associated with the type of cervical radiculitis that Carmen came in with. C2 tested that it needed to have energy moved **out**, and that the energy to be moved was associated with the flower essence Black-Eyed Susan, and related to the period of time when Carmen was 11 years old.

Black-Eyed Susan is not one of my favorite flower essences. Its character is about avoidance of painful aspects of the personality. This usually means that the patient has emotional energy that needs to be moved, but has it locked up tightly. Translation: they're in denial.

Carmen was an excellent example of this. She was a lovely, literally beautiful, woman who appeared to be the matriarch of her family. She was impeccably dressed, spoke articulately about herself and her physical symptoms, and obviously had a very close relationship with her adult daughter, Lissette, who was sitting with us in the treatment room. Carmen was the epitome of "a lady": regal, refined, emotionally controlled. I couldn't help sighing, reluctantly, as I reviewed the explanation of Black-Eyed Susan in the *Flower Essence Repertory*.

> **Black-Eyed Susan is a powerful catalyst for confronting parts of the personality or traumatic episodes from the past that have been kept locked away in the recesses of the psyche. Often these unclaimed parts of the psyche operate as shadow parts of the personality; for example, a person who was raped or abused may begin to exhibit the same behavior toward others later in life. In other instances this enormous repression does not manifest outwardly, but inwardly, in self-destructive tendencies or as mental or physical illness. In many cases Black-Eyed Susan is indicated for individuals who suffer from emotional amnesia and paralysis, and are totally unaware of the healing issues they must confront. What is needed in these circumstances is an increase of awareness; the ability to shine the light of consciousness into the shadows of the psyche. A great release of energy is felt in the soul once such buried parts of the psyche are consciously encountered and addressed in an appropriate therapeutic environment. Black-Eyed Susan restores great light and conscious awareness, helping the soul to integrate and transform unclaimed parts of the psyche.**

I gave Carmen the structural explanation for cervical radiculitis: localized muscle spasm causing a distortion of the normal alignment of the cervical vertebrae, with resulting nerve irritation and pain. She nodded her understanding, and I continued. What I wanted to know was why, exactly, did the muscles spasm? What was the trigger? She had no idea. She commented that she often had neck "tension", but never this severe, nor lasting so unrelentingly long. Stress, maybe?

A nice umbrella diagnosis, stress, but not actually specific enough to be helpful.

I explained that, according to my muscle testing, Carmen did have emotional stress stored in her neck; specifically, emotional stress from when she was 11 years old. I asked her to close her eyes and relax, take a couple of deep breaths, and let a picture come to mind that was about her 11-year-old time. To her credit, Carmen was very willing to cooperate, but she had the typical innocent-skeptic look on her face. Something like, "Who, me? Stressed? At 11?" She lay there several minutes, breathing deeply, while I worked on some of the muscle points related to her neck symptoms. Then I asked her to tell me what happened when she was 11.

She started out slowly, saying that she hadn't really thought about this in a long time. I could see her searching through her mental files, doing the math. She said she couldn't remember anything particularly interesting from that time. "Good," I said, because I actually didn't want her to "remember," I wanted her to "imagine." Memory is usually like a snapshot, an inanimate picture that's held in the mind. Way too intellectual for my purposes. Imagination is much more multi-sensual. You can imagine movements, textures, smells, etc. Most fun of all, you can also imagine feelings. I asked Carmen to imagine that her 11-year-old self could step into the private space of her own, adult imagination—as if she were walking into a room that exists only in Carmen's mind's eye. I asked her to notice, if her 11-year-old self were to show up in that room, how she would present herself: what would she wear, how would she have her hair, and more importantly, how would she be feeling, what would she be thinking? Carmen became very still as she worked at imagining how her 11-year-old self would appear if she were present right now. I waited quietly, until I began to see the tell-tale signs of Carmen's eyes flickering back and forth beneath her eyelids. She smiled ever so slightly, as in recognition of something so long ago seen that it's almost forgotten, when I asked her to describe what she perceived there.

She had a clear picture in her head of her 11-year-old self at boarding school. She could see her there, alone, and hating it. She felt completely isolated. She had been very close to her little brother before being sent away to school, and she missed him terribly. She felt very confused; she didn't understand why she was sent away. It felt like her world was ending, as though she had done something terribly wrong, and was being punished for it.

I asked her to let herself feel that. Feel how alone and abandoned she felt. I told her it was important to go all the way in to the feeling.

She cried. I'm pretty certain she rarely cried in front of anyone, certainly not a stranger. Nor her daughter. She cried the pain of her 11-year-old self, who probably never felt safe enough to cry. As I mentioned earlier, this kind of emotional release comes like a storm; it looks very dark and menacing, like something dangerous and uncontrollable, so we resist it. We avoid feeling the feelings because they look like they will overwhelm us; but like the thunderstorm, when we finally move into our feelings, or when we finally let the emotional storm overtake us, we just get wet.

It rains. Sometimes it just rains, and rains, and rains. There's thunder and lightning. It gets dark and windy, and when the clouds descend on us we can't see anything but where we are. Everything around us disappears into the inundating rain.

And then it's over. The storm fizzles out, the thunder disappears into the distance, and our normal world appears once again.

Gradually the energy of loss and fear dissipated. Carmen opened her eyes and smiled at me; a little embarrassed by her emotional display, but cognizant of the fact that her catharsis signified something important. I asked her if she had ever found out why she'd been sent away to boarding school.

Yes, she said, because after about six months away, she was allowed to return home. There she found that her mother, who had been widowed a few years before, had remarried. Apparently, her mother needed to get the children out of the way in order to pursue a courtship with Carmen's new stepfather, so Carmen was sent to boarding school, and her little brother was sent to stay with relatives.

Emotions are held in the body in connection with beliefs, and because emotions are the territory of the subconscious mind, the beliefs that are held with them are not necessarily logical. In Carmen's case, the belief that held all that rain in her body was that she had been sent away to boarding school, abandoned, because of something that she did. Something wrong. The release of a limiting belief from the subconscious mind can be achieved by bringing the belief to the attention of the conscious mind. The 11-year-old had formulated the belief—based on her circumstances, and her limited ability to understand them—that she had done something wrong. The belief then gets filed away in the subconscious mind, and in the body. The child-Carmen assumes that the painful experience was her fault, perhaps because questioning her mother's reasoning feels too dangerous: at that young age Carmen's survival was still very much dependent on her mother. The conscious adult-Carmen has many more resources—and much more wisdom—available with which to re-evaluate this belief, and its actual relevance to her current, adult circumstances. Understanding the belief, she can choose differently.

As I adjusted Carmen's C2 vertebra, I asked her to focus on releasing the belief from her body, as well as her 11-year-old self's body, that she was responsible for her mother abandoning her. Then I asked her to choose a different belief about what happened to her when she was 11, based on her adult understanding. She said that she had never realized how painful those six months at boarding school had been for her, but she did realize that her mother hadn't sent her because she had done something wrong. She knew that her mother had wanted to re-marry in order to give her daughter and son a father. And her mother had actually done a good job, because her stepfather was extremely loving toward her and her brother, treating them like his own children. She was grateful for the structure and the harmony he had brought to her home, and her life. She could easily believe, now, that her mother had sent her away to boarding school not to punish her, but rather as a misguided attempt to help her.

Excellent. Then she could also replace the emotion of fear and loss that had been stored in her neck with something less painful, and hopefully more productive. I cradled the C2 vertebra in my fingers, and asked Carmen to invite energy into it. I asked her to think about the emotions that she had just released from that area, and then notice the emotions that were available to replace them. I told her to choose which emotions she would like to have held in this bone, based on her new belief about what happened at 11.

She chose love. She sort of blurted it out before I could even finish my instructions. It was, after all, the logical choice. She took some deep, voracious breaths and drew in the energy of love, concentrating it into the spot where I held my fingers. With each breath, her own energy seemed to expand, as is wont to happen, under the influence of love. She couldn't help sighing, happily, when she finished.

Unable to leave well enough alone, I asked Carmen what she had been referring to, at the beginning of the session, when she asked me if "stress" could be the trigger behind her neck muscle spasms. She explained that for the past couple of weeks her eldest daughter, Lourdes, along with Lourdes' two young children, had been staying in Carmen's home. Besides the normal stress of having long-term houseguests, and small children in the house after so many years, there was a lot of emotional tension at home.

Lourdes was pregnant with her third child, and had recently found out, through some routine pre-natal testing, that the baby had some kind of congenital problem, which might need to be treated with a very sophisticated surgical procedure very soon after birth. Lourdes lives in a very small town in Europe, where this type of surgery is not available, so she had come to stay with Carmen through the pregnancy until the surgery could be performed. The doctors here in the States were running all sorts of tests now, in order to determine the exact nature and extent of the baby's problem.

Carmen was very naturally worried about her daughter, and the baby, but she realized now what had triggered her muscle spasms. There had been much talk at home about sending her two grandchildren back to Europe, where their father had to stay in order to work. The father was very lonely without his family, and did not want to be without his children for so many months. In addition, Lourdes was rather overwhelmed with the stress of the pregnancy and the impending birth and surgery. Carmen was very worried about how her grandchildren were going to feel, being sent away from their mother, and had been lobbying her daughter and son-in-law to allow the children to stay in her home during the process, in order to be with their mother. But the decision had apparently been made by the parents to send the children back to Europe. This had brought all of the unreconciled emotions of Carmen's own childhood right up to the surface of her subconscious mind. Until this moment, however, they had not reached her conscious mind.

I pointed out to Carmen that her grandchildren were very lucky to have her around, because she now knew how important it was to talk to them about their situation, to reassure them about how much they are loved by their parents, and to make sure that they had a safe space to process their own emotions. She could create that safe space for them, probably better than anyone, because she knew from experience just exactly what they needed; someone to talk to them, someone to listen to them. And what a magnificent opportunity for her own self-healing! She had a chance to give her grandchildren the exact thing that she didn't get as a child, when she was sent away from her mother. That kind of opportunity is just too synchronistic to ignore, or to waste.

If we are looking at **WHEN** energy to be moved *in* to the patient, we may be pulling in energy that originates from another time or, subtly different, moving energy in to a specific aspect of the patient that is *of* another time. Let's look at an example of both.

CASE STUDY #13 – CARMEN: Part II

I saw Carmen for a follow-up approximately a week after her original visit. She told me that her neck and arm pain had improved greatly, but that she was still feeling a deep "ache" in the upper back, between the shoulder blades. Muscle testing showed that the cause was at the spiritual level, and indicated that the heart (ORGAN) wanted spiritual energy moved *in*, with both WHEN and WHO qualifiers. The WHO was someone not currently in human form, and the WHEN was 7 years of age.

I tracked down the "person not currently in human form" to be best described as an "angel". This suited Carmen's cultural and religious framework very comfortably, so I knew it was a good label to use with her. For people with different spiritual orientations, a different term might work better, such as "spiritual energy", or "an aspect of the Higher Self". Using the right words, in the appropriate context, is very important; if in doubt, I muscle test different options until I find the one that works best for my patient.

So what Carmen's heart needed was energy to be sent in from her "angel" to nourish the 7-year-old aspect of herself. I asked Carmen to call into her mind's eye the 7-year-old, in the same way that she had brought in her 11-year-old on the last visit. But this time, I wanted her to look at how the little girl was feeling, in her heart.

Carmen described her 7-year-old as a classic tomboy. She was always on the go, getting into things, mostly into trouble. The little girl felt that she was "bad", because that was what she was constantly being told by her family. Her heart was filled with both sadness and frustration, because she had no idea how to be "good". Everyone else seemed to know, except her.

Fine reason to call in an angel. I asked Carmen to imagine the angel approaching her 7-year-old, to notice how this angel presented itself. Carmen was getting pretty good at going along with my odd requests, so she didn't even blink at this, just took a long, deep breath and let her imagination bring up an angel. I'm pretty sure that Carmen was preparing herself to visualize some benevolent looking woman with long flowing robes and golden hair. What she saw was her father approaching her. Her father in his work clothes, smiling at her.

Carmen explained that her father had died when she was just 4 years old, of a heart attack.

I gave Carmen a few minutes just to take in the presence of her father, then I asked her to tell him that we needed his help; to teach the 7-year-old how to be "good". I instructed Carmen to watch, and take note of what information her father would give the 7-year-old about how to be good. Carmen literally held her breath, waiting. Then she began to weep, very softly.

He's not saying anything to her. He picked her up, and held her, and just...just told her with feeling. No words.

Told her what?

*You **are** good.*

You are good. What a perfectly simple, and incredibly nurturing thing for a child to hear. Carmen continued, saying that her father then turned to her, the adult Carmen, and again without words, told her

Everything's OK. You are not alone.

Carmen broke into full-on tears at this point.

As I held my hands over Carmen's heart, one in front and one in the back where her pain had been when she came in that day, I told Carmen to take the energy of that statement in to her heart. To take the love of her father into her heart. To take the innocent goodness of that 7-year-old into her heart. Carmen gladly pulled it in, again breathing deeply and allowing her energy to expand.

It was in the intense focus of that moment that my intuition kicked in. I suddenly knew that we needed to send that same energy to the heart of Lourdes' baby, the little unborn child who was the center of so much emotional turmoil. I gently told Carmen that we were going to send that same feeling she got from her father into the baby's heart; to let it know that it, too, is OK, and that it's not alone.

We both set our intention on radiating the energy to the baby, breathing fully and letting the waves of feeling roll outward to find the heart of that little child, waiting to be born. The minutes ticked by in silence, laden with love, until we both somehow knew that it was complete.

I adjusted Carmen's spine in the areas that are neurologically related to the heart, wanting to set the energetic adjustment into the physical body. After that, Carmen explained to me that during the past week, since our last visit, the test results had come back to show that the baby had a hole in its heart. Surgery would be performed to repair it just 3 days after the birth.

Yeah, OK. Intuition's good.

I encouraged Carmen to take some time each day to send the same energy to the baby. I didn't need to point out to her, at that point, the power of energetic healing.

Carmen called me a couple of weeks later, and left me a message saying that she was feeling fine, thankyou for everything, and that she had decided to accompany her two grandchildren back to Europe until their mother returned with the baby.

In Carmen's case, we needed to pull in energy to nourish the 7-year-old aspect of herself. In other instances, as follows with the case of Stephanie, however, I might need to pull energy in from a younger aspect of the patient, to nourish her current, adult self.

CASE STUDY #14 - STEPHANIE

Stephanie had recently come through a rather traumatic divorce, and came to me because she was having difficulty getting herself "back on track" with her life. She didn't really have a clear sense of the direction that she wanted to head in, either professionally or personally, and she was feeling a distinct lack of focus.

Muscle testing showed all levels of the field involved, and led me to Stephanie's pancreas, (ORGAN) which was looking to move energy *out*. The qualifiers on the energy to be moved out indicated that it was related to the flower essence Aloe Vera (WHAT), as well as to her (WHEN) 10 year old self, and that it needed to be moved to (WHERE) her left lung (ORGAN). We also needed to look at WHY the left lung needed the energy.

Note that the pancreas is the organ in the body whose job is to regulate the blood sugar. At the energetic level, the pancreas is in charge of holding and processing the energy that is related to our sense of "sweetness" in life; our thoughts and feelings about life being sweet - satisfying and nurturing - or about where the source of that sweetness lies. The lung is the organ that regulates the most fundamental nutrient of life, air - our life force, the breath. Energetically the lungs are in charge of holding and processing our thoughts and feelings about loss, grief, and disappointment. So Stephanie's pancreas needed to give some energy to her left lung. The left side of the body is generally regarded to be the feminine side, and so is related to all things feminine; our intuition, our sense of home and nurturing, as well as any feminine people in our life – mother, sister, daughter, female friend. I knew that over the course of the past 2 years, Stephanie had not only divorced, but divorced because she found out that her husband was having an affair with one of her female friends. She had also lost her sister, who died suddenly of a brain aneurysm. And add to all that, the fact that soon after she had married her now ex-husband, her mother died of a heart attack. It was understandable that her left lung would need an infusion of "sweetness", after processing so much loss and grief.

 I had Stephanie relax fully on the table, and bring to mind an internal picture of her 10-year-old self, while I stimulated the pancreas reflex point. Stephanie grew up on a small island in the tropics, so she immediately saw her 10-year-old self sitting out in the yard of the house she had grown up in, enjoying the lush tropical landscape. Stephanie explained that she had been a very shy, quiet kid at that age (two words that absolutely no one would use to describe her now, by the way), and her house had often been filled with turmoil because of frequent arguments between her mother, father, and grandmother. When things became too chaotic for her, she would just go outside and sit, soaking up the calming energy of nature. I asked Stephanie how she knew, at just 10 years old, how to do that; to draw in the energy of nature and let it nourish her, calm her. She shrugged, as if everyone does that all the time.

The next step was to send this 10-year-old's energy, and I would assume her ability to heal herself with calming natural energy, into Stephanie's left lung. But first we needed to look at why the left lung required this energy. I looked up the *Flower Essence Repertory* description of Aloe Vera, the essence associated with the 10-year-old energy, in order to get some kind of a clue. It reads as follows:

Those needing Aloe Vera "burn the candle at both ends." They have an innate abundance of fiery forces, but tend to overuse these forces and literally "burn out." Typical of the Aloe Vera type are "workaholics" whose drive is so intense that they neglect their emotional and physical needs, often sacrificing rest, food, and social contact in order to accomplish their goals. Such an attitude cripples the ability to experience life in a heart-felt way, impoverishing the feeling life, and draining the body of vital energy. While will-power can carry such persons quite far, eventually they reach a point of exhaustion, burnout, or breakdown. Aloe Vera helps the soul and body aspects to come into greater harmony, by bringing the nourishment which comes from the water polarity of life – the flowing qualities of renewal and rejuvenation. When the soul learns to balance the fiery forces of the will with the fountain of feeling from the heart, a tremendous outpouring of positive creativity and spirituality can be realized.

This was one of those instances where the pieces of the puzzle didn't quite fit together. I couldn't see clearly how to link Aloe with the traditional lung issues, or with Stephanie's 10-year-old. And my intuition was giving me nothing. Blank. So, without reading the Aloe description to Stephanie, nor confessing my lack of insight, I simply—humbly—asked Stephanie to focus on the energy of her left lung area, notice its qualities, and then inquire of the energy, in whatever way seemed appropriate to her, why it needed the 10-year-old's energy from the pancreas.

I worked the lung points on Stephanie, front and back, while she took her time exploring the left lung energy thoroughly in her mind's eye. A couple of times she interrupted her breathing with a sigh, and I thought she was about to speak up and tell me what she had found in her internal expedition, but she just went silent again, breathing deeply and rhythmically. Finally she opened her eyes and said just one word.

Heat.

She said it somewhat apologetically, as though she thought she should have come up with more information, but that was all she had. In light of the Aloe Vera description, that was enough.

As I held one hand over the pancreas point, and the other over the left lung, I asked Stephanie to allow the calm, nature-nurtured energy that her 10-year-old self held to flow into the heat of that left lung. I asked her to pay attention to what happened when the two energies met. She took a few long breaths, allowing the energies to merge, and immediately responded that the left lung energy got cooler. She felt it relax her, calm her, relieve an anxiety in her that she hadn't even been aware of.

I encouraged Stephanie to practice this little visualization, as her own personal healing ritual, on a daily basis. This was the way she could nurture herself – be her own source of "sweetness". By taking a little time away from the chaos around her, she could give herself the energy she needed to focus on her life, and her future.

The "HOW" Qualities:

The appearance of the **HOW** qualities emphasizes the need for the patient to use her own perceptive abilities in order to become consciously aware of the qualities of the energy to be moved. I ask the patient to notice, as I did with Stephanie, how the energy appears in her inner perception. Everyone perceives energy a little differently, and each of us has a predominant sense that we tend to use first when perceiving energy. Some of us are kinesthetically oriented in our perceptions; we sense best through touch, tactile feeling and movement in our body. I think this is my strongest sense, as I often get a very physical sensation in my solar plexus area, my "core", as to the nature of an energy. It may feel hot or cold, vibrant or stagnant, rough or fine, tight or soft. Some people are more visual; they "see" energy, even if only in their mind's eye. They see color, form, shape, size. Some of us are primarily auditory. We hear the energy, sometimes as a tone, sometimes as a word or series of words. Occasionally, I see patients whose main sense it olfactory. They smell the energy. Whatever sense, or combination of senses, we use to perceive the energy, it's all good; it informs us.

If we are moving energy *in*, I will ask the patient to perceive how the energy presents itself, and then watch how it influences the body's own energies as it enters. If we are moving energy *out*, I first ask the patient to perceive the energy as it sits in their body, and to notice its effect, both on their body and on their being. The patient's perception is important here, because things are not always as they seem. Such was the case with Annette.

CASE STUDY #15 - ANNETTE

Annette had been working with me for a few sessions already, and we had moved a lot of her physical symptoms out of the way by gradually uncovering the fact that, in spite of being an enormously successful professional woman, she was holding back her gifts.

Everyone has a gift. Some of us have a few, and some people's gifts are more dramatic than others, but everyone has at least one gift. We can move through life without ever realizing what our gift is, we can be aware of our gifts but never develop them, or we can develop them without ever putting them to good use. We can function perfectly well in these cases, and even, as with Annette, be successful, in the traditional definition of the word. But we cannot be happy. You have to use your gift in order to be happy, at least according to my observations.

Annette came in to do a session centered on the question of why she holds back her gifts. Interestingly, Annette had never asked for my assistance in determining the nature of her gifts, implying that she already knew, but neither had she given me any indication as to what her gifts were. Muscle testing indicated that the reason for holding back these gifts was an energy pattern at the mental level of the signature energy, and located in the fifth chakra, where energy needed to be moved both *out* and *in*, in that order. The mental energy pattern to be moved *out* was qualified as being associated with her 2-year-old self, as well as with the flower remedy called Self Heal. In addition, we needed to look at the HOW and the WHY of this energy.

I asked Annette to breath deeply for a few moments, allowing herself to relax and "go within". I instructed her to allow a picture to come up and into her mind's eye that was about her 2-year-old time, just noticing the first thing that came to her mind. She saw herself in the house that her family moved into just about the time she turned 2 years old. She explained that her parents had purchased the house, which had two stories, and then remodeled it before they moved in. During the remodeling period she and her siblings had lived with their grandparents, so she felt very happy when it came time to reunite with her parents. However, she felt very uncomfortable in the new house.

Her parents had taken the open loft configuration between the first and second story and closed it in, extending the second floor out into the area that had previously been open to a high vaulted ceiling above the first floor living room. Of course as a 2-year-old, Annette had been too young to understand these details. All she knew was that there had been a "hole" in the floor, and now it was covered up. For some reason, this scheme of things resulted in the terrifying belief that she would fall through the floor of the second story if she strayed beyond the boundaries of what had been the "hole in the floor".

I asked Annette what would happen if she fell through the floor. Immediately her body seemed to contract inward, as if she was becoming very small, and she answered me in the soft, hesitant voice of a frightened child.

I would disappear.

Disappear to where? Where would you go?

I don't know. Somewhere else. Somewhere bad.

The fear of falling is one of the fundamental instincts of the human/animal body. Two years old is certainly old enough to be aware of the normal consequences of falling – that is, the sudden impact of landing. And yet, this was not Annette's concern when it came to falling through the "hole". It was not being hurt that she feared, it was "disappearing." This was my first indication that Annette had something unusual going on. Where could this belief have come from? I asked her to focus her inner vision on the energy of the fear of falling through the hole in the floor. I wanted her to perceive how that fear energy presented itself, from as many levels of perception as she could use. I encouraged her to see how it looked, hear how it sounded, or what it said, and notice both how it felt to touch it, and how it made her feel.

It looks like concrete...like a concrete block. It's a pressure. It presses on me and makes me feel like I can't move.

I told Annette to ask the fear energy why it was pressing on her; what was its purpose, or intention toward her. Normally, I would expect the answer to be something like "protection", since this concrete block of fear seemed to be preventing Annette from falling through a dangerous (at least from the point of view of her 2-year-old mind) hole in the floor. If this were the case, it would be a fairly simple job for her adult-self to explain the reconstructed floor reality to her 2-year-old, so she could then release the belief that she could fall through, thus releasing the need for the protective restriction of her fear. This could also easily have explained why Annette had difficulty moving into new and unfamiliar places, something that is often required when it comes to sharing one's gifts. Perhaps she was afraid of going outside of familiar boundaries for fear she would "fall through" and then "disappear"—lose her identity.

Her answer surprised me.

Possessing. It wants to possess me.

She said it out loud, after a long and apparently excruciating hesitation, in a tone that conveyed just exactly how much conflict she felt about such an idea. Everything in her body language now said, "Please, just don't tell me I'm crazy".

Far be it for me...

But how *does* one interpret such a statement? The fear wanted to possess her: this certainly makes the "disappearing" take on a whole new meaning. Is it possible that there were non-physical entities in residence in Annette's new home, and that these entities wanted to "possess" her? Can it be that the "hole in the floor" was some kind of energetic vortex, which led to an alternate reality that was home to these entities?

Or could we say, just to tone it down a little, that the 2-year-old Annette believed that the reality that existed under that hole in the floor was completely separate from her own, and that if she stepped into it, she would not be able to find her way back? Certainly we could conclude that the fearful beliefs she held about falling through the floor were needing to be discarded, or at least reformed, and were somehow related to her reluctance to express her gifts.

We went about the business of moving this fearful mental energy out of Annette's fifth chakra. I asked her to use her intention, and her breath, to gather up this energy, this concrete-like pressure in her throat that wanted to possess her, and push it out. Out of her body, out of her field. I worked on the muscular trigger points in the area while she breathed, and then released the pattern from the body with an adjustment of the C5 vertebra, which is energetically related to the fifth chakra.

Next we needed to look at the energy to be moved *in* to this area. It's interesting to note here that the energy that normally flows outward from the fifth chakra is about self-expression, which makes this chakra a good place to work on Annette's issue of holding back her gifts. Obviously the fear energy that we had just released from the area had been an impediment to self-expression. Moving energy in to the area would hopefully replace the fear with something more conducive to good "gift usage."

My muscle testing indicated that the energy to be brought in was also related to Annette's 2-year-old self, and required that we again examine the WHY of the energy. I asked Annette to return to her 2-year-old, noting that the little one was holding something for her: an energy that could now be brought in to replace the fear energy that we had removed. I told her to focus on the energy that the 2-year-old held, and see what sense she could get of the purpose of the energy, and why the 2-year-old was holding it.

She has this power...I have this power...to go into your dreams.

Annette shook her head and flung her hands out, as if waving it off, like she wanted to take it back as soon as she said it. She blushed with embarrassment, explaining that it seemed silly, but it was the only thing that the 2-year-old had to say.

It's not silly, I assured her, but certainly a talent that only a young child could accept without questioning. She agreed, saying that such an idea was considered very strange, and even dangerous, amongst the adults of her little world.

I continued, mentally noting that it sounded like Annette had a gift for out-of-body travel. I asked the 2-year-old why she went into people's dreams. She again returned to the shy and delicate body language of a young child, looking for the right words.

Just...To hold your hand.

Ah! A guide. A spiritual guide. Annette apparently had a gift for spiritual guidance that she had been holding back because of fear. Fear of "falling through the hole" and disappearing, losing her identity, being possessed – whatever those things really meant. At any rate, it was our job to bring that gift back in to Annette's adult consciousness, from its storage place in her 2-year-old. Once again I asked Annette to breath deeply, this time drawing the innocent acceptance of the child in to her fifth chakra, reclaiming the knowledge and the power of "going into dreams".

Later, I lent Annette a copy of one of Robert Monroe's books on out-of-body-travel. I also went in to my flower essence collection to find a bottle of Self Heal for her to use at home. My usual procedure, when dispensing flower essences, is to pull the appropriate bottle from the display shelves in my "pharmacy", and make a photocopy of the page in the *Flower Essence Repertory* describing the essence. The flower essence bottles are lined up on the shelves alphabetically; this makes finding them easier since I keep several dozen different essences in stock. I followed this procedure with Annette, pulling a bottle of Self Heal from the shelf, and moving to the photocopier to copy the Self Heal page. As I was waiting for the copier to warm up, I glanced down, and noticed that the bottle in my hand was not Self Heal, but another essence entirely: Mountain Pennyroyal. This was very odd, because I was certain I had pulled the bottle from the row marked "Self Heal", which is not even close to the Mountain Pennyroyal row. It was almost as if the Mountain Pennyroyal had "jumped" into my hand, insisting that I give it to Annette. When I remembered the characteristics of Mountain Pennyroyal, which are described below, I decided to give her both essences.

Hygiene is as important to the life of the soul as it is for the physical body. Mountain Pennyroyal particularly addresses an individual's mental field which may be devitalized due to psychic congestion from too many negative or chaotic thought forms. There can also be mediumistic tendencies in such persons, so that they unconsciously absorb the negative thoughts of other persons or entities. When developed to an extreme state, the individual may no longer be able to think clearly for him/herself, or make rational decisions. There may be a tendency to possession, especially if the person is prone to using alcohol or other drugs. In these cases, seemingly conscious actions are actually carried out at the behest of others' intentions rather than those of the true Self. Mountain Pennyroyal works as a purgative; it has the powerful ability to cleanse and expel negative thoughts, or the unhealthy intrusion of entities in the astral body. This essence clarifies the mental body and leads to greater vitality of the mental life, especially positive, clear thinking.

CHAPTER 10

THE QUALITY OF WHY

The primary motivation for me to develop Signature Energy Work was the directive from my college days: to bring healing and love to people. A lot of years have since come and gone, and I think I can honestly say that, back then, I had very little idea what I was talking about. The true motivation behind Signature Energy Work, I have since come to understand, has been to create a mechanism for exploring the true meaning—*my* true meaning—of love, and healing. Signature Energy Work is the tool that I have used for self-inquiry, both in resonance with my patients and on my own; for self-discovery: bringing my unconscious premises up to the light of consciousness; and for self-creation: creating a revised set of operating premises based on a higher level of truth. In short, for my own self-healing work. If it doesn't work for me, I can't expect it to work for anybody else.

And so now we come back to my little cold from Chapter 6. If you recall, I had already found out that the energy involved with my cold was from the mental level, located in my heart, and needing to be moved *out* through my sixth chakra. The energy was of the character of the flower essence Goldenrod, and required that I examine WHY it was there, before I could move it.

When the energy quality "**WHY**" tests positive, I use, as my energy-work modality, a method that is based on the Core Transformation techniques. These techniques are described fully by Connirae and Tamara Andreas, in their book, *Core Transformation*[47]. (I encourage you to read this book thoroughly and master its techniques.) You will find a more detailed description of my version of "Why Processing" in Appendix F.

Before I started moving my "cold" energy, I read what the *Flower Essence Repertory* had to say about Goldenrod:

> *Our earliest sense of Self unfolds within the context of others – parents, extended family and community. Gradually, through a healthy maturation process, the soul acquires a clear sense of its individuality. Some souls do not successfully complete this individuation process, remaining too subject to group mores, and family ties. These souls need to establish their own inner values and beliefs, otherwise their inherent weakness is easily exploited. They tend to be adversely influenced by social pressures and conventions, conforming their behavior to social norms in order to win approval and acceptance. In some situations such souls will also display antisocial or obnoxious behavior as an extreme measure to acquire a self-image – this is especially true during adolescence. Goldenrod essence helps such persons to find a true relationship to the Higher Self. It encourages a vertical or individuated axis to counterbalance the overly broad, horizontal social axis, which influences the personality too strongly. In this way the soul acquires greater strength and inner conviction, learning to successfully balance the polarities of Self and Other.*

With this in mind, I close my eyes, breathe deeply to relax and go within, and focus on the energy that is around my heart. It looks yellow and thick, with streaks of red (and the gross similarity to the current state of my sinuses is not unnoticed). I let myself be surrounded by this energy, allow it to swirl around me so that I can feel it at all levels, and send out a mental request to it, asking it to tell me why it has been in my heart. What is its purpose, for me?

I "sense" that it wants to protect me.

Good, thank you for that, but what is that protection supposed to do for me, exactly?

Allow me to be "loose".

Loose—I let the feeling of the word flow over me. I recall my swim team days, in those moments before a race, when all the training and 5 AM workouts come down to one full-self hurtle off the starting block. The last moment before the starting-gun sounds is all about loose. Loose with an explosion of energy held in potential. And what was the "looseness" meant to do for me?

The word "uninterrupted" floats up. So the potential held within the looseness needed to be uninterrupted. Uninterrupted in order to—what?

"Independent."

OK, the energy held within the looseness needed to be uninterrupted so that I could be independent. I like that; I'm desperately independent, but I have often wondered why I feel compelled to be *so* independent. I tend to go too far, and stray into isolation, so I have to be careful. I have been trying to master that delicate balance for years. You definitely have my attention, now. What *is* the purpose of this independence?

I find my imagination pulled into a scene where I am standing in front of a magnificent, full-sky sunset. The colors of yellow with streaks of red again surround me, but this time in the form of a sunset so breathtaking that I feel my heart expand joyfully, trying to take it in. I feel myself standing on the rocks of a high precipice, taking in this desert sunset, dressed in traditional Native-American medicine-man clothing. I am so tuned in to the natural energies of the Earth, the Sun, the Sky, that I *am* the sunset at that moment. I feel the depth and breadth of the ancient wisdom that I am connected to in this sacred place, in this sacred timeless moment, and I am inundated with a sense of reverence. The exquisite feeling of pure, natural power expands with every breath and brings me to a vibrational crescendo that is nothing short of absolute awareness. Full presence.

It takes me what feels like hours to come back from that place, although it is probably just a matter of moments in real-time. As the image and the rush of feeling dissipate, I ask again: Why?

It occurs to me that I need to be independent in order to safely tap in to the beautiful, ancient knowledge represented by this medicine man's connection to the sunset. This makes perfect sense to me, because the society in which I was raised doesn't honor this type of ancient knowledge, or its power, at all. But why me? Why do *I* need to connect with this knowledge? What am *I* supposed to do with that kind of power?

"Teach".

The energy of this word is strangely peaceful. Like the focused looseness of the athlete surrounds and feeds the raw power of her physical strength, the peaceful energy of Teacher embraces and holds within it the vast power of all knowledge; the wisdom of the higher Self.

So as I understand it, my cold is about discharging (literally) and releasing the negative energies of Goldenrod, which are the restrictions/limitations placed on my individuality by my family, or more specifically, and ever so redundantly, by the primary holder of my family persona, my mother. This, in order to unlock the positive energies of Goldenrod within me—the true nature of my Self. Myself as the Teacher. In order to write this book, to allow myself to be so bold as to make a public statement of what I think I know, I must see myself, in some form, as the Teacher. I have to release the pattern from my signature energy that is about being unable to, or unworthy of, holding that kind of power.

The operative word, I think, is holding. I cannot, in the smallness of my normal (imperfect) human life, even pretend to *be* that powerful. But I can act as a vessel for that power, a channel if you will, for the wisdom and knowledge of my Higher Self, the Teacher. And in the process of acting as the vessel, holding the higher wisdom and knowledge for my students and my patients, I can actually glean of little of that knowledge and wisdom for myself. And that, as they say, is the key to the kingdom.

CHAPTER 11

STEP FOUR -- RE-TEST

Once I feel that the energy moving process is completed, that the energy is fully transformed and the new energy pattern is fully integrated in to the patient's consciousness—the patient "gets it": they fully understand the nature of the problem pattern as well as their own part in creating it, and they have chosen a new pattern based on that awareness—then it's probably time to move on. We may need to move on to another issue or another location, or we may be ready to wrap it up and move on with our day. I like to re-test to be sure there's nothing we've missed by asking the following questions:

IS THIS LOCATION COMPLETE?

If no, then we need to find out what else is required in this same location, by asking

DO WE NEED TO MOVE MORE OF THE SAME ENERGY?

A "yes" answer to this question would imply that we didn't move the energy fully, and so need to go back and continue our energy-moving in the same way (with gusto).

A "no" here implies that we need to move a different type of energy in the same
location, which would mean returning to the SEWLINE questions.

If the location is, in fact, complete, then we would want to know:

IS THERE ANOTHER AREA THAT WE NEED TO WORK ON TODAY?

If yes, you will need to return to the SEWLINE and ask about a new location.

If there is no other area to be worked on, move to STEP FIVE.

CHAPTER 12

STEP FIVE: THE EPILOGUE - PROCESSING, HOMEWORK, AND REFERRALS

We shall not cease from exploration
And the end of all our exploring
Will be to arrive where we started
And know the place for the first time.
      - T.S. Eliot

   When the energy-work is complete, the patient (and the practitioner) are often left feeling a little "altered". It is important to make sure that everyone is grounded before moving back into the mainstream of everyday life, so I like to spend at least a few moments after the session "processing" what happened: what was the exact nature of the energy that was transformed, how did the energy work feel, what impressions did we get about what it all means, and where do we go from here? Signature Energy Work is an on-going process. It's a process of becoming conscious of our own energies: the nature of our signature energy, and how we use it. It's a process of raising our consciousness, our signature vibrational frequency, to continually higher levels. It's the process of individual evolution. As such, each Signature Energy Work session is cumulative; it works on the signature energy that is present in the moment, which is a result of the Signature Energy Work that has gone before. Not every Signature Energy Work session has a nice, neat ending. It can take several sessions to clear out a particular "issue," and issues tend to interconnect with other issues. I have been using the work on myself for years, and, believe it or not, I'm not perfect yet. But I know myself better, and I've come a long, long way from where I started. I believe Signature Energy Work is a lifelong tool for personal growth.

Signature Energy Work is just one tool, however; one that operates in synchrony with many others. The variety of healing modalities that are available to us in this modern life is vast, and Signature Energy Work functions in a complementary manner with almost every one. This is why I encourage my patients to continue their healing work when they leave my office, either in the form of "homework" or a referral for additional treatment with another type of practitioner.

Homework is something that I "assign" to the patient as a healing treatment or activity, to be performed by them, on their own time. This might be a meditation or visualization to be repeated on a daily basis, as was the case with Stephanie, who needed to practice using the energy of her 10-year-old self to calm and heal her body. Nancy's homework was in the form of a long-overdue conversation with her employer. I will often suggest a flower essence for the patient to take home and use regularly, reiterating the energetic intention of our Signature Energy Work session with each dose of flower essence.

Referrals to other practitioners, when appropriate, are a vital part of the patient's healing process. I often refer patients for acupuncture, nutritional counseling, psychotherapy, physical therapy, yoga, traditional medical care, and even other types of energy work. I consider Signature Energy Work to be just one spoke on the wheel of healing modalities, and I encourage the patient to be the "driver"—the centerpoint and director of his own healing and personal evolution program. When in doubt as to whether a particular homework or referral is appropriate, I ask - I muscle test on the question.

At the end of the session, when the energy-work is done, the homework and referrals are made, and it looks like everything is complete for the day, it's always good to approach the quantum self one more time, muscle-testing on the final question:

IS THERE ANYTHING ELSE?

After all, muscle-testing is where we started. It seems like a good place to end, for now.

NOTES

CHAPTER 1:
1. Braden, Gregg, *Walking Between the Worlds,* Radio Bookstore Press, Bellevue, Washington, 1997, p. *xiiii*.
2. Pert, Candace B., *Molecules of Emotion,* Simon & Schuster, 1999, p.146.
3. Hawking, Steven, *A Brief History of Time: From the Big Bang to Black Holes,* Bantam Books, New York, 1988, p.18.
4. Braden, Gregg, *The Isaiah Effect,* Three Rivers Press, New York, 2000, p.96.
5. Goswami, Amit, *Physics of the Soul,* Hampton Roads Publishing Inc., 2001, p.263.
6. A theory developed by Einstein in which electric, magnetic, and gravitational phenomena are treated as parts or phases of a single process. (*World Book Dictionary*)
7. Hunt, Valerie V., *Infinite Mind: Science of the Human Vibrations of Consciousness,* Malibu Publishing Co., Malibu, CA, 1989, p.20.
8. Ibid, p.66.
9. Ibid, p.111.
10. Braden, Gregg, *Awakening to Zero Point,* Radio Bookstore Press, Bellevue, Washington, 1993, p.30.
11. Goswami, Amit, *Physics of the Soul,* Hampton Roads Publishing Inc., 2001, p.13.
12. Ibid, p.43.
13. Reid, Daniel, *The Complete Book of Chinese Health and Healing,* Shambala Publications, Inc., Boston, 1994, p.271. (Reprinted by arrangement with

Shambhala Publications, Inc., Boston, www.shambhala.com)
14. Hoffman, Enid, *Huna: A Beginner's Guide,* Para Research, Gloucester, Mass., 1976.
15. Maslow, Abraham, *Toward a Psychology of Being,* John Wiley & Sons Inc., NewYork, 1998.
16. Collective reality is created from the perceptions of the collective consciousness. "In terms of collective consciousness, the developmental and spiritual literature describes an evolutionary progression, leading to ever widening circles of identification and care: from a particular group (marriage, family, organization, etc.), to a acommunity...to a society or culture...to all sentient beings, to Nature...to the globe...to the cosmos..." (from an online article by Robert Kenny, Ph.D., 2004)
17. Pribram, Karl H., "Holonomy and Structure in the Organization of Perception", Mimeographed, *Department of Psychology, Stanford University,* Stanford, CA, n.d.
18. Bohm, David, *Wholeness and the Implicate Order,* Routledge & Kegan, London, 1980.
19. Hunt, Valerie V., *Infinite Mind: Science of the Human Vibrations of Consciousness,* Malibu Publishing Co., Malibu CA, 1989, p.63.
20. Pert, Candace B., *Molecules of Emotion,* Simon and Schuster, 1999, p.310.
21. Ibid.
22. Goswami, Amit, *Physics of the Soul,* Hampton Roads Publishing Inc., 2001, p.45-46.
23. Hunt, Valerie V., *Infinite Mind: Science of the Human Vibrations of Consciousness,* Malibu Publishing Co., Malibu CA, 1989, p.56.

24. For example, see Brennan, B., *Hands of Light,* Bantam Books, 1987.
25. White, John, and Krippner, S., *Future Science,* Anchor Books, New York, 1977.
26. Brennan, B., *Hands of Light,* Bantam Books, 1987, p.43.
27. Palmer, P., *The Courage to Teach,* Jossey-Bass Publishers, 1997.
28. Ibid.
29. Resonance – the principle of physics that gives us the concept that "like attracts like", wherein a body that is vibrating at a certain frequency has that vibration reinforced by exposure to another body vibrating at the same frequency. In electronics, information is sent from a transmitter to a receiver, but the receiver must be tuned to the same frequency as the transmitter – be in resonance with it -- to receive that information.

CHAPTER 2:
30. For a clear (and illustrated!) explanation of O-ring testing, see Wright, Machaelle Small, *MAP: The Co-Creative White Brotherhood Medical Assistance Program,* Perelandra, Ltd., Jefferson, Virginia, 1990.
31. For a thorough discussion of muscle-testing, and the history of its use, see Hawkins, David, *Power vs. Force: The Hidden Determinants of Human Behavior,* Hay House, Inc., Carlsbad, CA, 1995.
32. Kendall, H., Kendall, F., Wadsworth, G., *Muscles: Testing and Function,* Williams and Wilkins, Baltimore, MD, 1971.
33. Diamond, John, *Behavioral Kinesiology,* Harper & Row, New York, 1979.

Diamond, John, *Your Body Doesn't Lie,* Warner Books, New York, 1979.
34. Hawkins, David, *Power vs. Force: The Hidden Determinants of Human Behavior,* Hay House, Inc., Carlsbad, CA, 1995.
35. Brennan, Barbara, *Hands of Light: A Guide to Healing Through the Human Energy Field,* Bantam Books, New York, 1987

CHAPTER 3:
36. Hawkins, David, *Power vs. Force: The Hidden Determinants of Human Behavior,* Hay House, Inc., Carlsbad, CA, 1987, p.246.

CHAPTER 4:
37. Goswami, Amit, *Physics of the Soul,* Hampton Roads Publishing, Inc., 2001, p.165.
38. Hoffman, Enid, *Huna: A Beginner's Guide,* Para Research, Gloucester, Mass., 1976, p.22.
39. Ibid, p.20.
40. Goswami, Amit, *Physics of the Soul,* Hampton Roads Publishing, Inc., 2001, p.122.
41. Mallove, Eugene, "The Cosmos and the Computer: Simulating the Universe," *Computers in Science* 1, No. 2, (September/October) 1987.

CHAPTER 6:
42. Hoffman, Enid, *Huna: A Beginner's Guide,* Para Research, Gloucester, Mass., 1976, p.21.
43. Newhouse, Flower, and Isaac, Stephen, *The 7 Bodies Unveiled,* Bluestar Communications, Woodside, CA, 2001, p.62.

44. Pearce, Joseph C., *The Biology of Transcendence: A Blueprint of the Human Spirit,* Park Street Press, Rochester, VT, 2002, p.4.
45. Kaminski, Patricia and Katz, Richard, *Flower Essence Repertory*, The Flower Essence Society (a division of Earth-Spirit, Inc.), Nevada City, CA, 1994, p. 320. Used by permission

CHAPTER 7:
46. Braden, Gregg, *Walking Between the Worlds: The Science of Compassion,* Radio
Bookstore Press, Bellevue, WA, p. xiv.

CHAPTER 10:
47. Andreas, Connirae and Tamara, *Core Transformation: Reaching the Wellspring
Within,* Real People Press, Moab, Utah, 1994.

APPENDIX A: "O-RING" TESTING

Kinesiologic testing can be performed on any muscle, and is often used as a diagnostic tool in orthopedic and neurological medicine to evaluate the level of weakness of an injured muscle or a muscle innervated by a damaged nerve. In Signature Energy Work we choose a normal muscle to test on, and use it as a diagnostic tool to access and read the signature energy. Many kinesiologists muscle test using an arm muscle, most often the deltoid muscle, whose function is to raise the arm laterally. I prefer to use the adductor muscle of the thumb, the "O-ring" muscle, simply because it results in less work for both me and the patient during repetitive testing. Here's how it works: ask the patient to hold the tips of the thumb and pinkie finger of one hand together firmly, forming an "O" with the hand.

1. Test the normal strength of this muscle by attempting to pull these two fingers apart, using each of your own index fingers placed inside the "O" and pulling outward. Normally, the patient should be able to maintain the "O" against your pull. This is the "yes" mode to our question/answer process.
2. Ask the patient to hold the "O" together, and then silently ask to be shown the "no" mode, while again pulling outward on the patient's fingers with your own. A "no" answer is demonstrated when the patient is unable to sustain his thumb and pinkie held together against the pull of your fingers.

This should not be a life or death struggle between you and the patient, so instruct the patient to hold his fingers together firmly against your resistance, but not to throw his whole body into it. Your resistive pull should be firm also, but not so firm that you are always pulling the patient's fingers apart. You may have to go back and forth a few times, asking to be shown "yes" and "no", in order to get a feel for the patient's muscle, and to find the right amount of pull you need in order to make a consistently clean test on that particular patient. Each patient is different, so play with it a little.

If the patient is not at all able to hold his fingers together, because of injury to the hand, overall weakness, inability to comprehend the muscle test mechanism, etc., or if you are unable to register a "no" response with the patient, you may have to choose another muscle to test against, or move to surrogate testing (see Appendix D).

APPENDIX B: FUNNEL TESTING

When we are testing over a large volume of information, we can use funnel testing to cover a lot of territory in a short amount of time. I use funnel testing the most is when checking for flower essences, so I'll use that as an example to demonstrate how funneling works.

If, during the course of my SEWLINE testing, it is revealed that a flower essence is to be used, I locate the specific essence by first asking if one of the flower essences that are in my collection (which is held in a small cabinet in my treatment room) is the one needed. If this tests positive, I can proceed to narrow the focus gradually, first asking if the flower that is needed is in the 1st drawer of the cabinet, the 2nd drawer, etc., until I find a drawer that tests positive. I then narrow the focus again by asking if the flower that is needed is in the 1st row of that drawer, the 2nd row, the 3rd, etc., until I find the row where the flower is positioned. I then test each bottle in that row, until I locate the one bottle that tests positive. My cabinet has 6 drawers, each drawer containing 3-5 rows, and each row holding 4-12 bottles (depending on the size of the bottle). The process of funneling down from a few hundred bottles to just one takes less than a minute.

This process is also useful for narrowing down periods of time, collections of homeopathic remedies and herbs, geographical locations, etc.

APPENDIX C: SURROGATE AND SELF-TESTING

Surrogate testing can be performed by using another person to muscle test on as a stand-in for your patient. I often use surrogate testing when examining small children: I ask an adult (usually the mother or father) to hold or embrace the child/patient while I muscle test using the adult's hand muscle, but asking questions about the child. This is usually great for two reasons: small children tend to be intimidated by strange doctors, and are often too young, or too squirmy, to focus on sustaining a muscle-testing mode for more than a minute or so.

I also use myself as a surrogate for my patients when necessary. This requires mastering the fine art of muscle testing on one's self. I usually do it like this:

1. Form the "O" with the thumb and pinkie of your non-dominant hand (for right-handed people, the left hand is non-dominant).
2. Use the thumb and index finger of the dominant hand to push apart the "O".
3. If you can push open the "O" with your other hand in response to a question, this registers as a "no" response. If the "O" stays closed, this is a "yes" response.

Self-testing means using yourself as a surrogate for yourself. Follow the above 3 steps, while asking questions about yourself as the patient. This is the key to using Signature Energy Work as a self-care modality.

APPENDIX D: GROUNDING AND CONNECTING

If you are a body-worker—your style of energy work involves physical touch—I
t is imperative to be grounded while you are working. Like it or not, when you touch someone in a healing mode, you are entering the boundaries of their signature energy, and resonating with it. You will pick up some of their energy in this exchange, and unless you know how to ground your energy, and to dissipate the other person's energy that you have absorbed by channeling it out through your grounding mechanism, you are going to end up wearing a lot of other people's energy, and eventually end up with physical illnesses and all the signs and symptoms of burnout. In addition to this, when you are doing healing work that involves the more subtle layers of the energy field—the emotional, mental, and spiritual levels—your grounding is what allows you to be aware of your patient, and his or her physical needs, while you are working with their emotions, thoughts, and beliefs. I like to ground with the following procedure, but there are many other great ways to go about grounding, so please find a grounding routine that works for you, and use it regularly.

1. Bring yourself fully into your physical senses. Take a moment to look around you, and fully **see** what you see. What does the space around you look like, and how does your patient look. Take a good, long deep breath and come fully into your own eyes.
2. **Listen**. Notice the sounds that are around you, pay attention to what your patient is saying, or to the rhythm and depth of his breath. Take a deep breath and come fully into your ears, your jaw, your neck and your throat.

3. **Feel.** Feel the position and tension in your own body, in your hands, your arms, in your torso, and your legs. Bring your body into a nice, relaxed, balanced position. Breath fully into your chest, your back, your belly, your legs and feet.
4. Bring your seeing, hearing, feeling, your intention and your breath downward from your feet and into the Earth. Sense your energy moving downward through the Earth to its center, and connect there. Take a moment to see, hear and feel the energy of the Earth; the compassionate intelligence that is the Earth. Breathe your breath fully down into the Earth energy. Release any leftover, unwanted energy that might be hanging around in your body down through this channel that you have created between your body and the Earth's center, and surrender it. Give it over to the Earth to be recycled into fresh, new, life-giving energy.
5. Take a hearty breath-full of the Earth's life-giving, rejuvenating energy, and return up the channel, back fully into your body. Now you're ready to work.

Connecting - to your spirit, to your Source – is so profound and extensive a subject that it would be absurd for me to think that it can be explained, or even should be explained, within the confines of one small page. It's a lifelong study. That said, here are the symbols and intentions that I use to focus on that connection.

1. Focus your attention on the spirit connecting point between your 7th and 8th chakra. This is the point that is directly over your head, approximately 3 feet above you.
2. Breathe your energy upward from the top of your head, through the energetic portal that is your 7th chakra, and

SIGNATURE ENERGY WORK

        toward that spirit connecting point above your head, and connect there. Feel, see, and hear the energy that you connect with at that point.
3. Surrender any dissonant energy that may be in your body up and out through the connection point.
4. Breathe the pure, bright spirit energy down through the connecting point, in through your 7th chakra, and down into your body.

Remember that the work of moving energy on your patients requires that you be grounded **and** connected, at the same time.

APPENDIX E: WHY PROCESSING

I use this technique to explore the WHY of energy; its purpose.

1. Ask the patient to connect with the energy involved, in the way that feels most comfortable for them, in order to "talk" to the energy, and find out it's purpose.
2. Instruct the patient to acknowledge that this energy has a purpose that is, at least from the energy's point of view, for the benefit of the patient. So, with gratitude, have the patient to ask the energy what that purpose is. What is it that this energy is trying to get the patient to experience, or understand?
3. Give the patient a few minutes to allow an answer to come to mind. If this seems slow in coming, gently remind the patient that the energy may not communicate in words, but rather in pictures, symbols, or just feelings. Encourage the patient not to judge what comes to mind, but rather just to notice it.
4. Take the answer that the patient receives, and interpret and clarify it, as needed, by asking the patient to take a moment to sit with the answer, and feel what feelings and/or thoughts come up with it. In Chapter 7, the answer that I received from my "cold" energy was that it wanted me to feel protected.
5. Once again, focus on the original energy, and thank it for pursuing that purpose, for your benefit. Then ask it this: if this purpose were fulfilled, and you actually did come to experience or know the thing that it was trying to get for you, what would it want for you next? Or, better said, what is the higher purpose of the energy that, by achieving the original purpose, it is trying to

lead you to? In my case, the protection was meant to help me to feel "loose".
6. Interpret and clarify this answer, as needed, and ask again, if there is a higher purpose beyond this.
7. Repeat this process until you and the patient are certain that you understand the highest purpose of the energy.
8. Feel this highest purpose. Ask the patient to explain to the original energy that he now understands the highest purpose, and because he understands it, it is no longer necessary for the energy to be there, trying to lead him to this highest purpose. The energy can then be moved and/or given a new purpose, of the patient's choosing. My "cold" energy was trying to get me to embrace my own archetypal Teacher. Once I understood this, and began to take initial steps moving in that direction, the cold could be released.

APPENDIX F: SEWLINE

LOCATION:
- Level(s)
  - All levels
  - Physical
  - Emotional
  - Mental
  - Spiritual
- Chakra
  - See Diagram D
- Organ
  - See Diagram E
- Body Region
  - See Diagram F
- Specific Body Structures

DIRECTION:
- In
- Out

BLOCK:
- Entry
- Exit

THE SIX W'S: (Can be applied to Directional Energy as well as Block)
- Who
  - Patient/Other
  - Individual/Group
  - Known/Unknown
  - Human/Other
- What
  - Color

SIGNATURE ENERGY WORK

        Homeopathic Remedy
        Flower Remedy
When
        Early Life
        Past Life
        Current Life
        Future
Where
        To
        From
How
        Seeing, Hearing, Touching, Feeling, Smelling
Why
        See Appendix F

APPENDIX G: SEWLINE REPORT OF FINDINGS

NAME: _____

DATE: _____

LOCATION:
    Level(s) _____
    Chakra _____
    Organ _____
    Region/Specific
Structure _____

OTHER QUALITIES:

DIRECTION						
In						
Out						
BLOCK						

SIGNATURE ENERGY WORK

	WHO	WHAT	WHEN	WHERE	HOW	WHY
Entry						
Exit						

RESOURCES

For more information on flower essences, contact:
Flower Essence Society
P.O. Box 459
Nevada City, CA 95959
USA
Mail @flowersociety.org
www.flowersociety.org

The Flower Essence Society is an international membership organization of health practitioners, researchers, students, and others interested in deepening knowledge of flower essence therapy. Founded in 1979 by Richard Katz, it was incorporated as part of the non-profit organization Earth-Spirit in 1982. Since 1980 the society has been co-directed by Patricia Kaminski and Richard Katz, who are married and professional partners. There are four major purposes of the Society: 1) to promote plant research and empirical clinical research on the therapeutic effects of flower essences; 2) to conduct training and certification programs for active flower essence practitioners, as well as public classes and seminars throughout the world; 3) to disseminate publications about flower essence therapy to practitioners and to the general public throughout the world; and 4) to provide a communication and referral network for those who are teaching, researching, or practicing in the field of flower essence therapy.

The *Flower Essence Repertory* was written based on the research and clinical observations of practitioners throughout the world.

For more information on kinesiology and self-testing, visit:
Perelandra Center for Nature Research,
www.perelandra-ltd.com.

The Institute for Advanced Spiritual Research,
www.veritaspub.com

For information on homeopathy, I suggest:
Consumer's Guide to Homeopathy, Dana Ullman, Tarcher, New York, 1995.

Materia Medica with Repertory, Wm Boericke, Boericke & Tafel, Santa Rosa,1927.

Emotional Healing with Homeopathy, Peter Chappell, Element, Rockport, MA, 1994.

For information on Signature Energy Work Seminars and Workshops offered by Dr. Cora Llera, please visit our website:
www.SignatureEnergyWork.com
Or call: (305) 672-2998

www.ingramcontent.com/pod-product-compliance
Lightning Source LLC
Chambersburg PA
CBHW030926180526
45163CB00002B/472